Taoist Secrets of Eating for Balance

Taoist Secrets of Eating for Balance

Your Personal Program for Five-Element Nutrition

Mantak Chia and
Christine Harkness-Giles

Destiny Books
Rochester, Vermont

Destiny Books
One Park Street
Rochester, Vermont 05767
www.DestinyBooks.com

Destiny Books is a division of Inner Traditions International.

Originally published in Thailand in 2017 by Universal Healing Tao Publications under the title *Five Element Nutrition: Secrets of Eating for Balance with Inner Alchemy Astrology*

Note to the reader: This book is intended as an informational guide. The remedies, approaches, and techniques described herein are meant to supplement, and not to be a substitute for, professional medical care or treatment. They should not be used to treat a serious ailment without prior consultation with a qualified health care professional.

Cataloging-in-Publication Data for this title is available from the Library of Congress

ISBN 978-1-62055-751-8 (print)
ISBN 978-1-62055-752-5 (ebook)

Printed and bound in the United States by Versa Press, Inc.

10 9 8 7 6 5 4 3 2

Text design and layout by Debbie Glogover
This book was typeset in Garamond Premier Pro with Futura, Present, and Sho used as display typefaces.
The following photographs are by Eve Lome and are used with permission: fig. 2.4 (right)—*Do Not Test,* fig. 4.1—*Plus loin s'en vont les secrets,* fig. 5.1 (both)— *Etre dans l'echec'* and *La force centripéte de la grandeur,* and fig. 6.1 (both)—*Cartes blanches* and *Autoportrait de son devenir.*

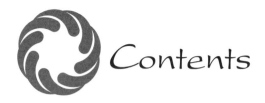

Contents

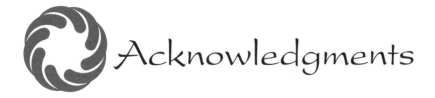

Acknowledgments

The authors and Universal Healing Tao Publications staff involved in the preparation and production of this book offer our gratitude to the many generations of Taoist Masters who have passed on their special lineage in the form of an unbroken oral transmission that extends over thousands of years. In particular we thank Taoist Master Yi Eng (One Cloud Hermit) for his openness in transmitting the formulas of Taoist Inner Alchemy and Juan Li for the use of his beautiful and visionary paintings that illustrate Taoist esoteric practices.

We offer our eternal gratitude and love to our parents and teachers for their many gifts to us. Remembering them (and the thousands of unknown men and women of the Chinese healing arts who developed many of the methods and ideas presented in this book) brings joy and satisfaction to our continued efforts in presenting the Universal Healing Tao System. Their contribution remains crucial in presenting the concepts and techniques of the Universal Healing Tao (UHT).

We are grateful and indebted to photographer Eve Lome for her unique five-element series, to Pavlo Maksymenko for his genius work in the Inner Alchemy astrology program, and to Josefine Reimig and Wolfgang Heuhsen for their support and organizational work for the Inner Alchemy astrology program within UHT Berlin.

Our thanks to Colin Drown for his editorial work and writing contributions and to our many instructors and students for enabling the years of research for this material and a true inspiration for this book—without them the book would not have come to be.

A special thanks goes to our Thai production team for their work on the original edition of this book—Hirunyathorn Punsan, computer graphics; Sopitnapa Promnon, photographer; Udon Jandee, illustrator; and Suthisa Chaisarn, production designer—and to the Inner Traditions editorial team for their abridging, simplifying, and rendering of the English of the original book to make it suitable for their American readership.

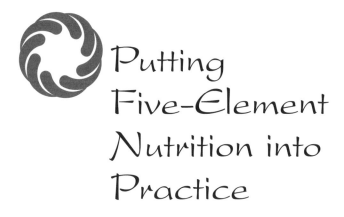

Putting Five-Element Nutrition into Practice

The information presented in this book is based on the authors' personal experience and knowledge of five-element nutrition. The practices described here have been used successfully for thousands of years by Taoists who have been personally trained in knowledge that has been handed down through an unbroken lineage of masters. Readers should not undertake the practices without receiving personal transmission and training from a certified instructor of the Universal Healing Tao, since certain of these practices, if done improperly, may cause injury or result in health problems. This book is intended to supplement individual training by the Universal Healing Tao and to serve as a reference guide for these practices. Anyone who undertakes these practices on the basis of this book alone does so entirely at his or her own risk.

The meditations, practices, and techniques described herein are not intended to be used as an alternative or substitute for professional medical treatment and care. If any readers are suffering from illnesses based on physical, mental, or emotional disorders, an appropriate professional health-care practitioner or therapist should be consulted. Such problems should be corrected before you start Universal Healing Tao training.

Neither the Universal Healing Tao nor its staff and instructors can be responsible for the consequences of any practice or misuse of the information contained in this book. If the reader undertakes any exercise without strictly following the instructions, notes, and warnings, the responsibility must lie solely with the reader.

This book does not attempt to give any medical diagnosis, treatment, prescription, or remedial recommendation in relation to any human disease, ailment, suffering, or physical condition whatsoever.

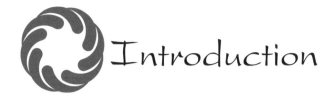# Introduction

The five elements could be understood as a comprehensive template that organizes all natural phenomena into five master groups or patterns in nature. Each of the five elements—wood, fire, earth, metal, and water—are also characterized by a description of a season, a direction, a climate, a stage of growth and development, an internal organ, an emotion, a taste, a color, and a sound. The five elements reflect a deep understanding of natural law, the universal order underlying all things in our world. Five-element theory developed over many centuries as Taoists laid out their ideas about cosmology. What an amazing system—the entire cosmos, from the macrocosm to the microcosm of the human body, can be understood in terms of the five elements and of yin and yang. These five elements are exactly delineated for each person by the position of the planets at the time of his or her birth as determined by Taoist astrology (which is Chinese astrology). This reveals so much about yourself, including how to best nourish yourself. This book considers this extremely important aspect of treating yourself well through nutrition, relating the Taoist theory of the five elements to your unique profile at the time of your birth.

Ancient Chinese texts written by Taoist masters describe the fundamental principles of nutrition. These basics involve eating locally grown, seasonal, freshly harvested foods. Although some of these principles are now frequently mentioned by modern nutritionists, in today's world, with its many technological advances, these ideas, which are actually very old, are rarely put into practice. Nowadays we can easily buy a variety of food flown in from all over the world (at the cost of a high carbon footprint). Non-native vegetables are often grown in countries where the inhabitants are struggling to feed themselves already, and then served up thousands of miles away. There are economic and gastronomic reasons for why this happens, but Taoist philosophy does not advocate any of them.

The reason locally grown, seasonal, freshly harvested foods are highly prized in Taoist philosophy is simple: this kind of food maintains the highest level of chi, or vital energy. Our Taoist forebears had no knowledge of whether foods contained vitamins such as C or K or E, but they did know what energy certain foods have available to those who consume them. The origin of all food is plants—plants predigest the cosmic life force energy and concentrate it within themselves. This is then taken into our body when we eat these plants. Or perhaps these plants are eaten by fish or other animals that we then later consume. The animals take the plant energy they have consumed and transform it to another kind of energy. The food chain could be even longer if the animal we eat was first consumed by another animal, which in turn ate plants, thereby giving it a different form of energy by the time the nutrients get to us. Food that comes from a fridge, freezer, or shelf (the worst is food from a can) has diminished chi, even though this is a common way of organizing our meals, living, and eating today. The essence of Taoist thinking about food concerns its chi, and indeed this is what Taoist five-element nutrition is all about.

Ancient Taoist texts describe foods as being "hot for the liver" or "cooling for the kidneys" or "too yin for the heart," and in this way food and how it nourishes us have been meticulously documented for five thousand years. We can translate this into Taoist terms by saying that warming or heating an organ is a yang activity, while cooling is yin. There are also foods that are considered neutral, neither yin nor yang. Today we talk about pH, or the acid/alkaline balance, which was not something that ancient Taoists measured, but they nevertheless understood and strove for a balance of yin and yang. Master Chia has worked with these principles for forty years and has transcribed them into easy-to-understand classification tables that describe the chi of a food according to the five elements. In addition to these classifications, Taoist nutrition involves eating conditions and looking after the body to achieve optimum digestion and therefore maximum well-being.

Relocating from Asia to the United States some forty years ago, Mantak Chia became exposed to the melting-pot approach of the many ethnic diets and fad diets that proliferate in the West. Comparing these to Taoist and Asian diets, he realized that it is vitally important that we look at the five-element energies people are born with, as well as their present lifestyle and condition of the body in order to understand and affect a food cure for various health problems. He considered Western ways of looking at what a body lacks nutritionally and compared these findings with a person's five-element profile and corresponding needs to achieve a balance of the elements, which leads to health. Master Chia spent ten years working out a nutritional program based on the composition of the five elements one is born with as determined by Taoist astrology, and he has been refining it for thirty more years. His five-element nutritional program ties in with Inner Alchemy practices such as meditation and chi kung and other Taoist arts, which he has devoted his life to teaching.

Chinese astrology defines the five-element makeup of a person using calculations based on the year, month, day, and time of birth. The five elements correlate exactly to the major organs, and in any given chart some elements will figure more prominently than other elements, therefore the corresponding organ energy would be stronger. This is the foundation that each person works with for the rest of his or her life, and if any imbalances or weaknesses in the natal chart are not identified and corrected as needed, the person's health and well-being will eventually be negatively impacted, or rather health and well-being will be played out according to that person's five-element energies. But we do have the option of trying to harmonize them, creating a more favorable health pattern. Considering your own composition of five elements allows you to refine your Taoist practices as necessary and apply five-element nutrition to bring more harmony into your digestion and your life.

In this book we will first look at some of the basic concepts involved in the Taoist approach to food, beginning with the digestive process. Then we will learn the basics of how to apply the five-element approach to eating using your unique astrological profile at the time of your birth.

Chapters 4 through 8 describe each of the five elements in detail and include at the end of each chapter detailed food lists that apply to the organs related to that element. These food lists as well as other relevant tables have also been placed in the appendices at the back of the book for easy reference when you are analyzing your own chart.

You don't need to know how to do complex astrological calculations to determine your five-element composition and therefore your five-element nutritional protocol; Master Chia has devised a simple tool that will do that for you at his website, **https://www.universal-tao .com/InnerAlchemyAstrology**. By inputting your birth data there, you will find your five-element composition at the time of your birth in the form of a pictogram that tells you which element energies are strong and which are weak. From there, as you will see in this book, you can begin to incorporate the principles of five-element Taoist nutrition.

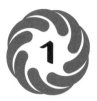

The Tao of Digestion

In the Taoist view, the five elements of earth, metal, water, wood, and fire are interconnected. In exactly the same way, the major organs that are associated with each of the five elements have to work together as a team to support the process of digestion. Let's take a closer look at this interconnected system.

Breaking down food—the start of digestion—has to start in the mouth with sufficient chewing; if this doesn't happen then it is more of a challenge to break down the food once it is in the stomach. As well, food must remain in the mouth long enough for it to be chewed to an acceptable pulp for the stomach to handle. The tongue has sensors in it that can feel the type and taste of the food it comes in contact with. It sends this information to the brain so that the correct digestive enzymes can be released into the stomach to help break down what is in the mouth and about to be swallowed and sent down to the stomach. Chewing is therefore a very important process in five-element nutrition, as the tongue's taste buds can identify the taste of the food it comes in contact with—and therefore the chi of the five elements—and determine which enzymes are needed to digest. So without proper chewing, digestion is impeded, creating more gas, making the passage through the large intestine difficult and painful. Yet more gas is produced as things become blocked, leading to constipation.

The pancreas and liver produce digestive enzymes and juices. The stomach mixes the food by pushing it around, like the drum of a washing machine, to break down the food and allow it to mix with the digestive juices. The worst scenario is when there is too much food in the stomach, and it's even worse if there is already gas there too. If your washing machine is too full of clothes, then the water cannot be mixed successfully to soak through them all properly and wash out the dirt. Similarly, the stomach needs at least one-third of its space to be empty to perform its action of properly mixing food and the digestive juices found in saliva. If this doesn't happen, then after trying to digest too much food the stomach will eventually send this mixture on its way anyway. Although at this point everything may be mixed together, the bile and other digestive enzymes cannot act properly on this poorly mixed substance. It nevertheless moves into the small intestine, which now feels uncomfortable because the nutrients are not in a free enough state to be absorbed properly.

At this point the digestion has become distressed and wants to push out the poorly mixed food. And because the digestion isn't working correctly, the blood cannot efficiently carry oxygen to all 27 trillion cells in the body. This is indigestion, and it can be so severe that it brings on illness. Another consequence of indigestion is poor absorption of the nutrients that we are paying so dearly for in our supposedly "great" diet!

So for good absorption of nutrients we need the stomach to send food on its way in a nano state, which is to say completely broken down. Otherwise nutrients cannot be absorbed first in the small intestine, and then in the large intestine. When this process malfunctions, it is in fact a form of malnutrition that affects other processes in the body: If there is not sufficient liquid in the large intestine, the stools will be uncomfortable to pass and the intestine will take water away from other bodily functions in order to try to do its job. The blood thickens, and the skin, the largest organ of elimination in the body, is deprived of sufficient liquid for toxins to be dissolved and eliminated through sweating.

This digestive stress continues with the lungs. If there is constriction in the large intestine there will be constipation, and this puts a strain on breathing, which can become irregular or labored. The lungs need to function well to take in oxygen and breathe out carbon dioxide. The large intestine, lungs, and skin are all metal organs, and any toxins present in these organs can prevent chi from circulating well. Constipation can even push on the diaphragm. Malfunctioning lungs, diaphragm, and large intestine form mucus, which can obstruct breathing, block the trachea and the throat, and further impede absorption of nutrients in the large intestine.

The kidneys and bladder function as organs of elimination, and poor functioning as a result of the impact of negative emotions will not allow them to eliminate properly. When you're relaxed, the bladder constricts and the kidneys can do their elimination work, as both are controlled by the vagus nerve; but under stressful conditions the bladder expands and the kidneys stop filling it with waste products, resulting in a buildup of toxins in the body.

THE FIVE ELEMENTS AS EXPRESSED IN THE HUMAN BODY

When studying the five-element model, it is important to realize that this multidimensional view of life offers a diagnostic framework to recognize where imbalances lie in the body, mind, emotions, and spirits. The five elements are precisely reflected in the major internal organs and the interconnected relationships between them.

The five elements are further linked to what in Taoist philosophy are called the Three Treasures, the fundamental energies that maintain human life. These treasures consist of universal or heavenly chi, higher-self or cosmic chi, and earth chi. All three are contained within the Taiji or yin/yang symbol. Traditionally, the Three Treasures are also visualized as three "palaces" or centers of the body, called the upper, middle, and lower *tan tiens*. The upper tan tien, which includes the third eye, the crown, and the entire head, connects to the universal chi through the force of *shen*, or spirit. The middle tan tien connects to the heart and other organs through the natural force of our soul, or *chi*, which is both the life force and the organizing principle flowing through all things and establishing our interconnectedness. The lower tan tien, located in the lower abdomen between the navel and the kidneys, connects the physical body, the sexual energy, and Mother Earth through the force known as *ching* (*jing* in Pinyin script), which gives cohesion to the physical aspects of life.

Strengthening and regulating the Three Treasures is one of the primary aims of Chinese medicine and five-element nutrition. When the Three Treasures are strong and balanced, we have mental, physical, and emotional strength. This leads to adaptability, a calm outlook, abundant energy reserves, and strong immunity. If we can reach this state, all aspects of life become easier. By balancing the organs through understanding our own five-element profile, we can also help balance the Three Treasures within ourselves. The following information about the organs associated with each element may give you insight into your own organ energy imbalances as well as meditative tools to bring them back into balance. Nutritionally you can use the insights you gain both from understanding the Taoist perspective of the yin and yang organs and from looking at the balance of elements in your basic chart to make food choices that will support your organs. However, if you would like to delve more deeply into how to create nutritional balance with the specific focus on each individual yin and yang organ, you can order more in-depth astrological charts or consult with a professional astrologer through the Inner Alchemy astrology portion of the Universal Healing Tao website.

The Fire Element

The heart and the small intestine are the main fire organs. The yin fire organ, the heart, is the lord, the commander of the person's psyche, the team leader and motivator. The shen, one of the Three Treasures, is associated within the heart and is at home in the upper tan tien, the heart area. It is the spiritual radiance that can shine from a person. It shows enlightenment, heart fire, and love and can be cultivated from chi and from kidney ching. The heart is a natural authority. It is a radiating, shining, brilliant energy. The heart communicates with the other parts of the body and the organs through the aorta and the arteries, with messages coming back to it from the veins.

As governor, the heart regulates the circulation and animation of life. It is at the center of the body, and without it nothing would work, as without the shen spirit there is no longer any life. If you have too much heart fire energy you must transform it into unconditional love, joy, happiness, and gratefulness; otherwise it will bring out impatience, hastiness, and even cruelty.

The small intestine, the yang fire organ, is responsible for receiving and making things thrive. Transformed substances stem from its fire. Energetically, in a yang and yin pair of organs, the yin organ is considered to be "full'" and the yang organ "empty." In the case of the fire organs the yang small intestine is empty with the capacity to both refill and to empty out. The heart can cultivate fire energy, and the small intestine can store it, to a certain extent. In terms of digestion, the small intestine fills and empties and sends on the digesting foods to the stomach.

The blood and blood vessels are also fire element. Good-quality blood is very important and affects our health in a major way, as witnessed by how we do blood tests as a basic measure to diagnose all sorts of health problems. Blood must be able to carry oxygen around the body properly, as every cell needs oxygen; therefore, the quality of one's fire and its associated emotions have a great impact on our lives. The body's currents, the blood vessels, radiate from the heart center. This demonstrates the radiating energy of fire and shows how this energy affects the whole body. If we stretched out all of the blood vessels and capillaries in our body, they could wrap twice around the equator. If you weigh twenty-five pounds more than your average weight, your heart has to work harder to circulate blood an extra five thousand miles.

The Earth Element

The pancreas, stomach, and spleen are the three earth organs, all vital to the digestive process. A yin earth organ, the spleen, stores and preserves all the nutrients that pass through it. The pancreas, also considered yin, manufactures hormones and enzymes needed for essential digestion. The stomach, the yang earth organ, is a storehouse for the distribution of those nutrients. These three earth organs work together as a team to circulate nutrients and the five tastes or flavors around the body to build up our blood, chi, flesh, and fluids.

The earth organs make up the middle heater, or tan tien, one of the Three Treasures, representing the junction of heaven and earth in human beings. These three organs must be strong to cultivate and store potentially available vital energy, chi. We can compare it to feeding the body with electricity; through Taoist Inner Alchemy practices, this form of energy can be transferred between the upper and lower tan tiens. The qualities that characterize earth energy explain why people with mainly this type of energy are good in construction, management, real estate, arbitrage, human resources, and so forth. Earth energy is slightly different from the other four energies. Directionally, it comes from the center, while fire, metal, water, and wood energies come from the four cardinal directions, south, west, north, and east respectively. In the seasonal cycle, wood, fire, metal, and water are associated with the seasons spring, summer, autumn, and winter (respectively), and the energies are vibrant during their own seasons. Earth is the "in between" seasons, the couple of weeks when the energies are in transition; for example, an "Indian" summer between summer and autumn. For this reason earth energy can sometimes resemble or mimic the qualities of the other four elements, and people with strong earth energy can apply that energy to many different skills.

The Metal Element

The lungs and the large intestine are the organs associated with the metal element, and the associated sensory organs are the skin and the nose.

Metal qualities include decision making, evaluating, and analyzing.

The lungs regulate the chi of heaven and earth. They govern life while acting on the orders of the heart, much like a chancellor or minister. The beating of the heart and the rhythm of breathing are interrelated. We often consider the heart and lungs as a working pair, and in this partnership the heart is regarded as yang and the lungs regarded as yin. They are such a pair that in transplant surgery they are often transplanted together.

Food alone is not enough to take care of the lungs; you also need good, clean air, and that means abstaining from smoking and from breathing polluted air. This points to the interrelationship between the lungs and the heart: when toxins are breathed in through the mouth and respiratory system, these can in turn block the blood vessels. A good cure for low metal energy is walking, as it increases your breathing, your lung energy, but it should be in a forest or by the sea where the air is good. In fact, before all the many powerful antibiotics were invented by the pharmaceutical industry, patients with tuberculosis were sent to mountain resorts for healing and recovery. It should be noted that advanced tuberculosis, a lung disease, negatively impacts the digestive system, with weight loss as a consequence, as there is an inability to use the nutrients in food—part of the job of the large intestine. This all demonstrates the interconnectedness of all of the systems of the body and all of the elements.

The Water Element

The water element is represented by the kidneys and bladder, both of which are essential for elimination, as well as the bones and the related sensory organs, the ears. Water represents strong will and purpose, clear ideas, and good feelings. The kidneys, the yin water organ, are responsible for creating power; skill and ability also stem from this organ. The kidneys contain the life force, and to this purpose they build up the marrow and the bones and create strength. Kidney energy is also related to sexual energy and to reproduction, the power of creative life force. The kidneys continually receive and store the essence of life. The ching essence, our primordial energy, is found in the lower tan tien, the kidney area, the store place of vitality. This is the physical energy of our very being that is necessary for sustained life. It is the most densely vibrating of the Three Treasures, but it can be lost through excessive ejaculation in men, heavy menstruation in women, and excessive stress, fear, and worry. We can rebuild our stock of it through Inner Alchemy practices and to a certain extent through diet.

The bladder, the yang water organ, is responsible for storing body fluids before they are eliminated. As with the fire element organs, there is a yin full organ, the kidney, and a yang empty organ, the bladder.

The world, the macrocosm, and our human body, the microcosm, are both about 70 percent water, so we always need to maintain a reservoir of at least 70 percent water. Imagine if you removed a significant amount of water from your body in such a way that you deplete this reservoir. When your water level drops, the thirst center in your brain is triggered so that you know you need to drink more water. When you're thirsty, you may experience all kinds of symptoms—headache, bad breath, dry skin, cramps, hunger, and general malaise. When this happens, you're not sick, you're thirsty. We often ignore our thirst response by not drinking enough. Many people avoid drinking water and substitute soft drinks and other highly sweetened drinks, or teas and coffee, which can be dehydrating. These drinks are usually not good for us and throw the whole system out of balance.

There are many brain problems these days, such as dementia and Alzheimer's, and a malfunctioning brain will give the wrong messages about eating and drinking. In addition, the body could be thirsty but the message comes across wrong, making an overweight person want to eat, which in turn requires more liquid to help with the extra digestion. The "sea of marrow," as the brain is sometimes referred to in traditional Chinese medicine (TCM), is just like a real tidal sea and needs to keep a backward and forward flow going.

It is commonly said that you should drink eight eight-ounce glasses of water a day; this will vary according to body weight. Although other drinks can count in this figure, you must consider what else is in those drinks; if there are toxins present in them you will need extra water to dilute and eliminate the toxins, which would not be counted in your basic daily water intake needs. Taking in large quantities of soft drinks, for example, will leave your thirst unabated and give your brain the wrong message that you have had enough to drink, whereas your body will need even more water to eliminate the harmful substances in those drinks. Recall the agony of thirst in "The Rime of the Ancient Mariner," by Samuel Taylor Coleridge: "Water, water, every where / And all the boards did shrink / Water, water, every where / Nor any drop to drink."

So make sure that you are quenching your body's thirst with suitable water.

The Wood Element

The liver and gallbladder are the wood organs. Planning and visionary energy is stored in the liver, the yin organ of wood. The gallbladder is the yang empty organ, and its function is to store the bile produced by the liver. If it cannot release bile regularly, then bile can build up to make bile stones, which in turn can impede proper functioning and lead to infections. If they cannot be removed safely, then the gallbladder might need to be removed altogether.

People with strong wood in their astrological chart are likely to be good at planning and organization and would use that energy well in life. If you have a lot of liver energy there are two things that can happen: either you become angry and frustrated, or you can transform that energy into kindness and generosity by doing the liver sound (see page 25) and smiling in generosity and kindness, and then sending it to the heart, turning it into compassion and love. Energy is always a two-way street—you feel your elements energy and you reflect it out so that other people feel this energy in you. People with a lot of wood energy would most likely suffer from jealousy themselves or make others around them feel jealous of them.

And you must use the energy in the right way or it can use you in the wrong way. Take the example of young people who are almost always very yang and have a lot of energy; if they don't use it for good they can use it for bad, from drawing graffiti on public walls to the much worse crimes of violence and terrorism. So for an excess of wood energy, you must convert it into kindness. Stress and anger affect your liver negatively. Before taking cholesterol medicine, try taking better care of your liver with Inner Alchemy practices and five-element nutrition.

HOW THE EMOTIONS IMPACT DIGESTION

We can see in the Taoist view that a human being's major organs hold the energies of the five elements of fire, earth, metal, water, and wood, and each of these elements has associated emotions, both positive and negative. Emotions play a huge part in digestion. As the Taoists say, holding anger and jealousy is like drinking vinegar. Indeed, these negative emotions of the wood element upset the balance of the wood organs, the liver and gallbladder, directly and in this interrelated system they also strongly affect the other organs, the hormonal system, and blood circulation. The vagus nerve transmits these emotions to the digestive system (and, of course, to other bodily functions too).

Let's consider how the emotions impact digestion, starting with the first in the cycle, fear, which affects both the kidneys and the liver. Fear is stored in the kidneys. If excessive, over time, this leads to a significant loss of energy, as our primordial energy, ching, is stored in the kidneys, which will eventually become depleted. As water feeds wood in the five-element generating cycle (explained in more detail later), the kidneys (a water organ) energetically feed the liver (a wood organ). So negative emotion of fear will be passed on from the kidneys, and then the negative emotions of wood, anger and stress, will produce malfunctioning in the liver. An overproduction of cholesterol can be a result of this. Nowadays, people are wary of eating fats because of various health concerns, particularly those that effect the liver, but they may not be looking at their lives and realizing that stress has the same negative consequences for the liver as eating the wrong kinds of fats do—in fact, stress may be even worse for the liver, as the jury is still out on the relationship between the cholesterol present in the blood and certain fats. Despite the differences of opinion, however, no health practitioner argues that too much stress is good for you.

Studies have shown that during periods of anger, jealousy, and envy, the gallbladder releases a lot of acidic bile, so the digestive juices emitted by the liver become very acid. The whole body then acidifies, and we experience a sour taste. This is particularly harmful if there is nothing

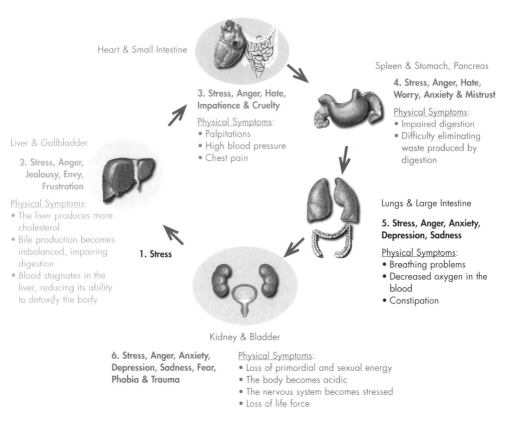

Heart & Small Intestine

Spleen & Stomach, Pancreas

4. Stress, Anger, Hate, Worry, Anxiety & Mistrust

Physical Symptoms:
• Impaired digestion
• Difficulty eliminating waste produced by digestion

3. Stress, Anger, Hate, Impatience & Cruelty

Physical Symptoms:
• Palpitations
• High blood pressure
• Chest pain

Liver & Gallbladder

2. Stress, Anger, Jealousy, Envy, Frustration

Physical Symptoms:
• The liver produces more cholesterol
• Bile production becomes imbalanced, impairing digestion
• Blood stagnates in the liver, reducing its ability to detoxify the body

1. Stress

Lungs & Large Intestine

5. Stress, Anger, Anxiety, Depression, Sadness

Physical Symptoms:
• Breathing problems
• Decreased oxygen in the blood
• Constipation

Kidney & Bladder

6. Stress, Anger, Anxiety, Depression, Sadness, Fear, Phobia & Trauma

Physical Symptoms:
• Loss of primordial and sexual energy
• The body becomes acidic
• The nervous system becomes stressed
• Loss of life force

Fig. 1.1. Stress, the emotions, and illness in the five-element cycle

to digest in the stomach, the acid will start working on the stomach walls instead. Acid indigestion is uncomfortable and a very common problem, as evidenced by antacid cures advertised on prime-time TV; such acid attacks can lead to ulcers and other problems.

Taoists long ago worked out which emotions affect which body organ through the theory of the five elements in as much as both positive and negative emotions are housed in the organs. Logically, if we want to use five-element nutrition, we must understand which emotions affect the body and how. Impatience and anger make the heart beat irregularly, which in turn causes high blood pressure. We might say that modern life causes a lot of today's illnesses, and that people living in earlier times did not have many of our modern, stress-related diseases, and they also had lower blood pressure overall. Today, anxiety, stress, worry, and impatience all impede digestion, starting with poor chewing of food in the mouth and moving on through the entire digestive route. Food does not look, smell, and taste good when digestion is hampered due to fear, worry, and anxiety. Frustration, which affects the liver and its ability to produce digestive enzymes, causes a lot of problems too.

Emotions, both positive and negative, are stored in the organs as shown in table 1.1.

Negative emotions are a leading cause of illness, so you have to really take care of your own emotional issues. If you are eating and you are angry or emotional, you generally will take the emotion into the stomach, and the whole digestive system will in turn become upset, even if you have a whole tableful of delectable food in front of you. An upset stomach is bad because it adversely affects the liver, and then no digestion can take place. In the West it used to be traditional to stop for a few moments before eating and say grace; this is actually a very good way to get rid of negative emotions and take a break from any premeal stress. You can then eat with a grateful heart. So although this custom is not as common now as it once was, saying grace or otherwise expressing a thankful, grateful heart helps us digest better.

TABLE 1.1. ELEMENTS, ORGANS, EMOTIONS, AND HEALING SOUNDS

ELEMENT	YIN ORGAN(S)	YANG ORGAN	POSITIVE EMOTIONS	NEGATIVE EMOTIONS	HEALING SOUNDS
FIRE	Heart	Small intestine	Love, joy, compassion	Hatred, cruelty, impatience, arrogance	Haw-w-w-w-w-w
EARTH	Spleen, pancreas	Stomach	Fairness, openness, trust	Worry, anxiety	Who-oo-oo-oo
METAL	Lungs	Large intestine	Motivation, courage, righteousness	Depression, sadness, grief	Sss-s-s-s-s-s
WATER	Kidneys	Bladder	Willpower, gentleness, fluidity	Fear and phobias	Choo-oo-oo-oo
WOOD	Liver	Gallbladder	Kindness, generosity	Anger, jealousy, stress	Sh-h-h-h-h-h

Almost every emotion affects the small and large intestines, the entire digestive system, and the body's ability to absorb nutrients. Worry and anxiety affect the top part of the intestines, and other emotions affect different parts of the digestive system and the body as a whole: fear affects the deeper, lower side of the intestines and the kidneys, and anger affects the right side of the abdomen by pulling on the digestive and absorption mechanisms.

The heart is the body's central intelligence agency, its CIA, regulating pulse and feelings and functioning as the nerve hub of the body (although there are actually more nerves in the stomach, and feelings are very buoyant there as well). Taoist Inner Alchemy practices can negate any upsetting emotions lodged in the heart. Forgive, forget, and release these negative emotions down into the earth. The earth can take our negative emotions and transform them into positive energy, in the same way that the soil can take our compost and use it to fertilize vegetables and flowers.

INNER ALCHEMY PRACTICES FOR DIGESTION

Inner Alchemy—the Taoist art and science of gathering, storing, and circulating the energies of the human body through certain practices—can help establish optimum digestion and absorption of nutrients, thereby contributing to overall health and well-being. Five-element nutrition and Inner Alchemy practices go hand in hand. Here is why:

The autonomic nervous system (including the vagus nerve and the parasympathetic nervous system) helps regulate many bodily functions: muscle movement, heartbeat, breathing, and especially digestion. It

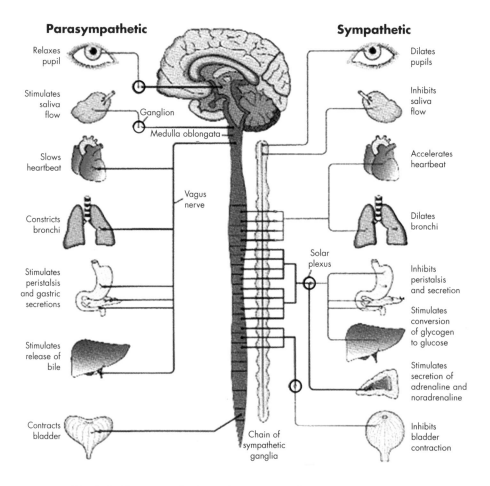

Fig. 1.2. The sympathetic and parasympathetic nervous systems

sends messages from the stomach to the brain and back again, stimulating digestive juices and contracting the intestine muscles to process and send food on its way.

Scientists have recently discovered what is considered another digestive organ, the mesentery, and although only recently identified as such, it was nevertheless featured in fifteenth-century anatomical drawings of Leonardo da Vinci. The mesentery connects the other digestive organs—the stomach, small intestine, pancreas, and spleen—to the abdominal wall, and it also seems to be involved in maintaining blood supplies.

The vagus nerve, the main nerve of the parasympathetic nervous system, is the longest cranial nerve in the body, descending from the head

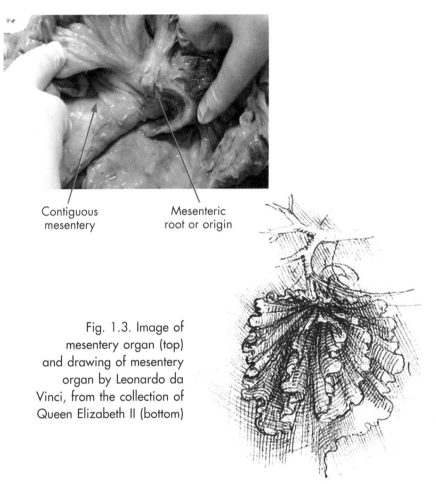

Contiguous
mesentery

Mesenteric
root or origin

Fig. 1.3. Image of mesentery organ (top) and drawing of mesentery organ by Leonardo da Vinci, from the collection of Queen Elizabeth II (bottom)

to the intestines. The parasympathetic nervous system has been dubbed the "feed and breed" and "rest and digest" reflex. It receives messages via the vagus nerve and puts the body's digestive parts into optimum digestive mode, stimulating the stomach, pancreas, and liver, thereby increasing the flow of saliva, bile, and other digestive juices. Stress and negative emotions constrict and tighten it, impeding good digestion, resulting in constipation, bloating, gas, and poor nutrient absorption. This will obviously negate any benefits that might accrue from following five-element nutrition principles or eating a well-balanced diet of healthy foods. This reaction to stress is the action of the sympathetic nervous system, which is responsible for the fight-or-flight reflex, making us ready to react to danger, but is counterproductive when we want to eat and digest, when we need to relax in order to do so.

By following basic Inner Alchemy techniques, we can relax the vagus nerve and allow it to do its job to the best of its ability. The Taoist Inner Smile meditation and the Healing Sounds, together with some basic chi kung movements such as crane neck and turtle neck, work well on this problem. Meditating on positive thoughts and smiling to create the virtues of the five elements will further optimize the body functions and eliminate obstacles to health and vibrant energy. Ancient Taoists studied life and health rather than disease and death, and these practices are designed to keep the body healthy and resistant to illnesses, so you can also think of them as disease-prevention techniques.

Ancient Taoist masters have long held that each of the major organs has an associated sound vibration according to their element (see table 1.1 on page 17). Recently, scientists have discovered that what actually distinguishes sounds from one another is their vibratory rate, and this may well explain how these internal exercises work.* The Healing Sounds combined with the Inner Smile are best practiced before bedtime, as they help cool down overheated organs, providing restful sleep. Some people

---

*For additional in-depth information on the basic Taoist practices described in this book, please refer to *The Inner Smile, Emotional Wisdom, The Six Healing Sounds,* and *Craniosacral Chi Kung.*

enjoy them during the afternoon to invigorate themselves if feeling tired or if they still have many things to do before the day's end.

The Inner Smile Meditation

Taoist sages discovered that consciousness is rooted not only in the brain but is found in every cell and every organ of the body. By literally smiling into the organs, thanking them for the work they do, we can reawaken the intelligence of the body. The Inner Smile meditation is often complemented with the Six Healing Sounds and is a simple and enjoyable practice for all ages, including children. (Note that only five of the healing sounds are used in this book as the sixth applies to the triple warmer, which is not included in this book as it is not connected to one of the five elements.) Traditionally regarded in China as an inner alchemy chi kung exercise, it seems to have originated among ancient Taoists, who were both philosophers and medical doctors. Just as we need good nutrition to nourish our physical body, we also need to nourish our emotional and spiritual bodies. The Inner Smile offers an excellent way to cultivate and activate the healing energies that are always around us. By adding color and sound to this meditation to activate and reenergize the body at a cellular level, this exercise is similar to many modern meditation techniques, yet more powerful.

The Inner Smile when combined with the Healing Sounds really gets results on the physical, emotional, and spiritual levels. Some people may find that at first using your mind's eye to visualize your internal anatomy is slightly difficult, but with regular practice it gets quite easy, even for those who struggle with creative visualization. Because your organs are actually in the place where you visualize them in your body and because they resonate with the colors and sound vibrations mentioned here, many will find this practice much easier than other visualizations; for example, a forest or some nice garden, images often used in modern creative visualization techniques. Visualization of something that does exist and is so close and personal, in this case the organs, which are actually inside you, is more natural and free-flowing.

Inner Smile Meditation combined with the Healing Sounds

We recommend doing the sound three times on each elemental organ in the order given and making the healing sound last until the breath is depleted before then breathing in the corresponding energy color.

1. Sit comfortably with a straight spine, either in a chair or cross-legged on the floor; the most important thing is that your spine is erect but free to move, and your neck is fully extended to allow the full flow of blood and energy up to your brain.

2. Close your eyes and begin to draw your attention inward. Listen to your breathing for several minutes as you inhale and exhale in a relaxed fashion.

3. Begin then to smile, but rather than smiling outward as you usually do in life, begin to smile back in, toward yourself. With your eyes closed and using your mind's eye (the third eye), visualize smiling back into yourself, as into a mirror. See your inner smile smiling back toward and into your body. We will bring the inner smile to each of the organs.

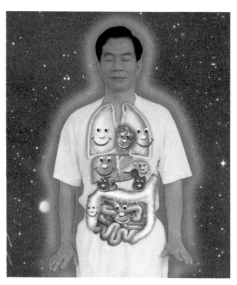

Fig. 1.4. Smile down into your vital organs.

❂ Metal Element
(Lungs and Large Intestine Sound)

1. See the left and right lungs in the chest cavity; they extend down to touch the liver and the spleen. The lungs are the center of energy cultivation and vital chi in the body. They regulate the opening and closing of the pores and also relate to skin health. Many of us use only the upper half of the lungs when breathing, being unaware of how far down they extend into the body.

2. The healing color of the lungs is pure white, the color of snow. Send this color into both lungs, seeing them being covered in the color white. Begin to visualize this color cleansing the lungs gently and smoothly. Eliminate any brown or black spots found there with this healing white light.

3. Once cleansed with the color white, make the sound *sss-s-s-s-s-s,* the sound of a snake, with your tongue behind your bottom teeth, while you are breathing out the negatives of metal: sadness, difficulty in letting go, and even depression.

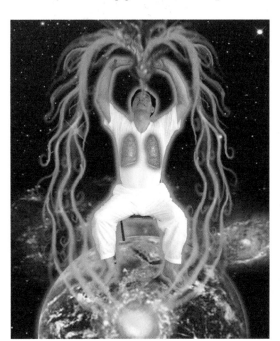

Fig. 1.5. Lungs and large intestine sound—make the sound *sss-s-s-s-s-s,* the sound of a snake, with your tongue behind your bottom teeth.

☯ Water Element (Kidneys Sound)

1. Focus on the kidneys, which are found along your midback. Feel the kidneys working, each day filtering all the body's wastes and regulating blood pressure and the acid-alkaline balance and many other duties that the kidneys perform each day for us.
2. Smile down into the kidneys, one on each side of your spine.
3. Visualize the color of the water element, dark blue, inside and around both kidneys. Using your imagination, clean the kidneys with the color blue, leaving no area unpainted with this color.
4. Once complete, make the sound *choo-oo-oo-oo,* and try shaping your lips as if you are blowing out a candle. You are breathing out the kidney or water toxins of fear when you do this. Then move on to the liver.

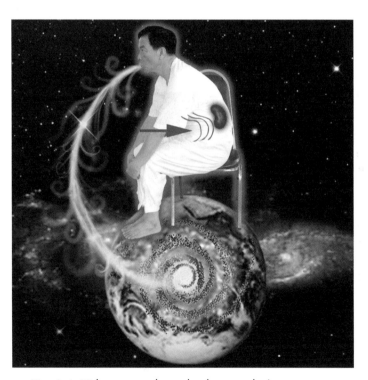

Fig. 1.6. Kidneys sound—make the sound *choo-oo-oo-oo,*
and try shaping your lips as if you are blowing out a candle.

☯ Wood Element (Liver Sound)

1. Visualize the liver, located under the right rib cage. The liver is a workhorse and needs regular attention in the form of positive energy and inner love. Smile into it. See it happily at work, cleaning your blood, producing bile, and regulating your metabolism.
2. Visualize the color green, as in the color of grass, and see the liver being bathed in this color. Use an imaginary paintbrush if you like to color it until it is completely green.
3. Seeing the liver bathed in green, make the sound *sh-h-h-h-h-h,* as you would if you were asking someone to be quiet, as you breathe out the negative emotions connected with wood: jealousy, stress, and anger.

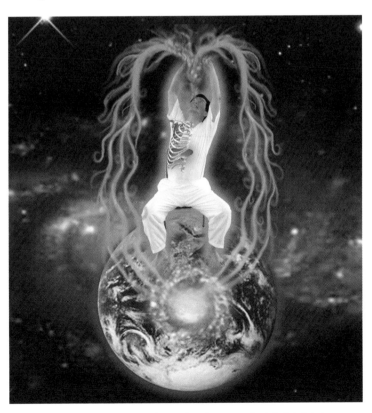

Fig. 1.7. Liver sound—make the sound *sh-h-h-h-h-h-h*
as you would if you were asking someone to be quiet.

☯ *Fire Element (Heart Sound)*

1. See your heart resting in the cavity of the lungs slightly left of center in your chest. The heart is the only muscle in your body that works twenty-four hours a day, even when you are sleeping or unconscious. It never rests and is fully functional up till the day you die.
2. Smile down into your heart and visualize the color red, the color of clean blood. See the heart bathed in the color red and being cleansed and nourished by this color.
3. Once complete, breathe out with the sound *haw-w-w-w-w-w,* like a deep, relaxing moan that originates from the chest rather than from the throat, as you breathe out impatience, hastiness, or any cruel thoughts.

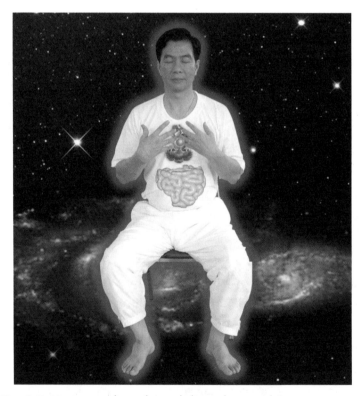

Fig. 1.8. Heart sound—make and direct the sound *haw-w-w-w-w-w,*
like a deep, relaxing moan that originates from the chest
rather than from the throat, into the heart.

☯ Earth Element (Spleen and Pancreas Sound)

1. See the spleen, pancreas, and stomach lying in the midsection of the torso toward the left-hand side under the ribs. These organs are directly related to digestion and assimilation in traditional medicine and to the element of earth, hence they are responsible for taking nutrients from food and creating the energy that supplies the other organs.

2. The healing color of these organs is yellow. Visualize the color yellow, like the color of a sunflower, and begin to see these organs bathed in this color.

3. Once these organs are cleansed in the color yellow, make the sound *who-oo-oo-oo,* originating in the throat, and breathe out the negatives of earth: unfairness, anxiety, and worry. Then breathe back in that wonderful yellow color and send it down into these organs.

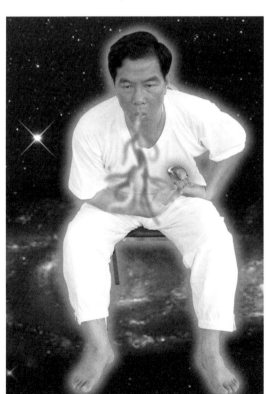

Fig. 1.9. Spleen and pancreas sound—make the sound *who-o-o-o-o-o,* originating in the throat, and breathe yellow light down into these organs.

In addition to these powerful Taoist Inner Alchemy practices, mindfulness practice is also extremely beneficial. Practitioners of this form of meditation are found all over the world, and their numbers are constantly increasing. Meditation and mindfulness have been practiced by Buddhists for thousands of years, and Taoist Inner Alchemy practices also use these tools. The bottom line is that we must take time out of our busy lives to meditate; otherwise there is no point in expecting any diet, miracle food, or five-element nutritional program to transform our lives and our health.

The Tao of Food

When we absorb chi from food it becomes our own chi. Chinese sages described this some five thousand years ago; they may not have known the scientific composition of food, but they did know that food contains vital energy, which affects our body and organs in certain ways.

When looking at nutrition we must consider how certain changes in the human diet and lifestyle have impacted our attitude toward eating and the level of chi available in food. Today we have greater food availability, but at the same time our food contains more sugar and bad fats than food did a hundred years ago. In addition, there were no genetically modified foods and other types of manufactured so-called foods. Because of the availability of all kinds of food these days, including food with little or no chi, we tend to eat things our ancestors rarely encountered. Another factor impacting our approach to food is the availability of formerly inaccessible foods. For example, whenever Master Chia visits Europe, he can't resist eating chocolate because the chocolate available in European countries is so good, yet until the 1600s, chocolate—a product of Central and South America—was unknown in Europe. In addition there is the matter of quantity: we eat so much more than what we need to eat in a day considering the decline in the average amount of physical labor we do today compared to what our ancestors did even only one hundred years ago.

THE ACID/ALKALINE BALANCE

The West may have discovered the importance of acid/alkaline (pH) balance in nutrition and other matters of health in recent years, but Taoist sages had already identified yin and yang facets of food (as well as all things of the living universe) thousands of years ago, saying that they must be in balance. This applies not only to our food, but to our saliva, blood, gastric juices, water, air, soil—indeed, to all matters pertaining to life. The Taoist idea of balance parallels the idea of acid-alkaline balance as defined by Western nutrition. Acid in this context means an acid-forming effect in the body, while alkaline refers to an alkalizing effect in the body. Though there are some differences between the two approaches, East and West, in general we can say that yin is alkaline and yang is acid. We need both acid and alkaline, both yin and yang.

Meats, sugars, pasta, grains, and processed foods are all classified as acidic, with some tap water and processed foods and meats being the most acidic of all. And a great assortment of vegetables and fruits are alkaline.

Acid, or yang, energy can be compared to the gasoline that fuels a car, while alkaline, or yin, energy can be compared to the oil needed to lubricate the parts of the car and thin down some of the glutinous, sticky fluids. Indeed, yin energy is necessary for the blood, joints, and connective tissue and for ensuring the flow and smooth working of the body.

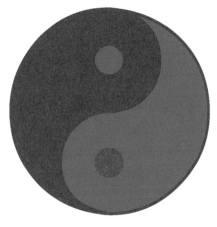

Fig. 2.1. The balance of yin and yang, a concept central to Taoism, parallels the concept of acid and alkaline.

Yin energy nourishes the body in order for it to save energy; it has a weight-losing effect and increases the energy input. Yang energy, in contrast, increases energy output, so a physically active job means you need a greater quantity of yang than you would need in a sedentary job. Both yin and yang together dictate how what we eat affects our metabolism—or rather the balance of the two does. As people get older and the level of their physical activity decreases, they obviously need less yang food. This change in the level of activity signals a change in the metabolism.

The Effects of Chronic Overacidity

Today the consumption of meat (as well as fast foods, sweets, processed foods, preserved foods, canned foods, liquor, all of which are acidic) is much greater than ever in the West, so in general our diet leans heavily toward the acid side. Add to that the effects of pollution and negative emotions, which exacerbate acidity, and we have a virtual epidemic of acidity. This is not so much the case in a few places in the world where relatively little meat is eaten, such as places that favor the Mediterranean diet or the traditional diet of the island of Okinawa, which relies chiefly on local vegetables and fish. But for the rest of us, acidity rules the day.

Too much acid in the blood is much more common than too much alkaline, and this can lead to metabolic acidosis, a condition in which the body uses its mineral reserves, such as calcium, as a buffer against all the excess acid. And when acid crystallizes in the arteries, mucous membranes, and joints, it creates inflammation and pain (gout being an example of this situation). In addition, stress increases acidity.

Two common problems that stem from metabolic acidosis are impeded digestion and constipation. With constipation, metabolic wastes are not properly removed from the cells, resulting in a clogging of the eliminative routes. This leads to even more acidity and toxicity, which in turn clogs up the large intestine. Once the mucous membranes are clogged, elimination becomes more and more incomplete, while the body becomes increasingly toxic, resulting in even more acidosis and a variety of problems such as heartburn, acid reflux, high blood pressure, cardiovascular damage, cholesterol plaque buildup, diabetes, osteoporosis, gout, arthritis, urinary tract infections, allergies, and asthma. There is strong evidence that digestion problems due to overacidity have a role in chronic fatigue syndrome and other forms of burnout as well. It is estimated that chronic acidity affects 95 percent of Westerners and is the culprit behind 90 percent of all human ills today.

In overly acid conditions the body becomes more and more polluted, while digestion becomes less and less efficient. We cannot acquire enough energy from what we eat, resulting in fatigue. The constant demand for energy that cannot be absorbed from food causes the metabolism to run amok and not work efficiently, further aggravating the condition. In addition, high levels of acidity (through the production of lactic acid) impede motor activity, which makes you tire easily when engaging in physical activity and can cause joint pain.

Excessive acidity has other associated problems. Negative thoughts arise and nightmares can occur, especially after overindulging in food and alcohol. Moreover, the liver has to work extra hard to filter out and remove the accumulated toxins, requiring large amounts of energy that are taken away from the rest of the body, contributing further to chronic exhaustion. The liver starts to produce more cholesterol while trying to clear toxins from the blood, a process known as chelation; this sends LDL "bad" cholesterol levels soaring, further contributing to the vicious cycle.

Obesity is another condition resulting from overacidification. The body creates fat cells to carry acids away from the vital organs so that these acids do not literally choke the organs to death, but these fat cells can nevertheless build up dangerously around the organs. Chronic overacidity corrodes body tissues slowly, eating into the approximately sixty thousand miles (that's 60,000!) of veins and arteries, the way acid can eat into stone or metal. If left unchecked, acidity will interrupt all cellular activities and functions, from the heartbeat to the neural firing in the brain. In short, overacidification interferes with life itself and leads to sicknesses and disease.

TABLE 2.1. NEGATIVE EFFECTS OF METABOLIC ACIDOSIS ON THE ORGANS

ELEMENT	ORGAN	EFFECTS
FIRE	Heart	Acidosis directly threatens the veins and arteries of the body and the heart itself, with added danger from higher blood cholesterol.
EARTH	Stomach and pancreas	Our body can respond to acidic conditions such as the risk of famine by overproducing insulin and accumulating fat. If the situation continues, diabetes can develop.
METAL	Lungs and large intestine	Digestion is impaired, and the large intestine stores more toxins, resulting in further acidosis. While trying to get rid of excess acid and toxins, the immune system deregulates, and mucous membranes start to produce more mucus, resulting in allergies and asthma.
WATER	Kidneys	The kidneys filter out the excess acid and eliminate it; this can result in kidney stones.
WOOD	Liver	Liver energy is depleted, so it works less efficiently, leading to exhaustion. To compensate and detoxify, the liver produces higher levels of LDL "bad" cholesterol, which attacks the heart.

In addition to its effects on the organs, acidosis contributes to arteriosclerosis, vascular constriction, and hypertension; it allows free-radical damage by attacking the nervous system and the DNA itself, leading to cell damage and premature aging.

It's easy to understand why we have such heavy acidity here in the West: these foods are so readily available. However, it's just as easy to compensate for acid-forming foods by including more alkaline-forming foods in your diet, which are also readily available. And that is just the point of the Taoist five-element approach to nutrition: balance.

Bringing Balance into Your Diet

Clearly we must prevent our blood, organs, and tissues from becoming too acidic; however, too much alkaline is not good either, so we must find a balance between the two. You cannot eat only alkaline; if your body does not produce acid, food cannot digest properly. If you do eat meat, adding vegetables to the meal makes the diet more balanced. But if you cook meat and vegetables separately and keep them apart on the plate—and even in the mouth, alternating mouthfuls of each—then they do not have a chance to mix well before the stomach phase of digestion. On the other hand, the fire and metal of cooking and heating meat and vegetables in a stir-fry will ensure that they do mix well.

In Chinese cooking the basic principle of adding some meat cut into small pieces and stir-frying it along with vegetables makes the acid-alkaline balance much better. The portion of meat in a single portion of stir-fry is less than what you would find in an average steak, which is commonly from 80 to 200 grams of meat—and we are not talking supersize here. That is a lot of meat for one person, especially if accompanied by fries, which are also very acidic. In addition, most Chinese dishes involve more than one flavor, such as with hot and sour soup, sweet and sour pork, and so on. Also we find most of the five-element colors in Chinese food. (More on color and flavor below.) We can do basically the same thing in other dishes—for example, it's fairly easy to make a five-element salad consisting of foods from all five groups, such as cucumber, sunflower seeds, cherry tomatoes, carrots, bean sprouts, seaweed, radish, corn, beets, and red peppers.

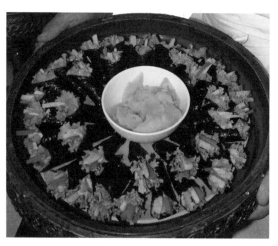

Fig. 2.2. Multicolored sushi dish

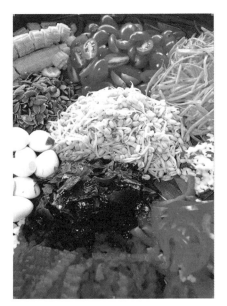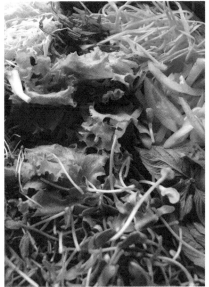

Fig. 2.3. Five-color, five-element salads

The traditional and much debated food pyramid indicates that 50 to 70 percent of our diet should consist of grains, 20 to 30 percent vegetables and fruit, and only 5 to 10 percent animal and protein foods. A good balance of food intake would be 20 to 30 percent acid food and 70 to 80 percent alkaline food. Growing children and adults under the age of forty may require the higher figures in the acid-producing foods. Adults over the age of forty should keep to the lower acid figures and the higher alkaline ones.

A general neutral acid:alkaline balance would be a pH of 7, and each bodily fluid has its own optimum pH, shown in this list of body fluids:

Bile, 7.6 to 8.6   Saliva, 6.35 to 6.85

Blood, 7.35 to 7.46   Semen, 7.2 to 7.6

Cerebrospinal fluid, 7.4   Urine, 4.6 to 8.0

Gastric juices, 1.2 to 3.0   Vaginal fluid, 3.5 to 4.5

Pancreatic juices, 7.1 to 8.2

The water you drink can vary widely in terms of its pH, with some common tap water being very acid. The average pH for normal drinking water is 6.6 pH, which is considered okay. You can measure the pH of your water at home so you'll know whether you are making your acid problem worse if the pH of your water falls under that figure. Alkaline water is between 9 and 11 pH; it neutralizes harmful stored acid wastes and gently removes them from the tissues. Reverse-osmosis water is almost neutral pH. Because of the extensive network of blood vessels in the body, there are many places where they can get clogged up, so it is essential that we maintain our pH balance. A good way to do this is by hydrating the body with alkalizing water. Food cravings are often the body's cry for water. A thirst for water will develop as one begins to hydrate with water.

As there has been increasing recognition that our diet has in general become so acid, there are now many exponents of diets that alkalize the body, and the growth in sales of alkaline foods cookbooks is an attempt to promote good health through dietary balance. But let us always remember that the body needs some acid, otherwise it cannot digest food and use the nutrients. The key is always balance, which is the heart of the Taoist approach.

THE FIVE SEASONS

The five energies, or the five elements of fire, earth, metal, water, and wood, are each associated with a season (see table 2.2). Fire correlates to summer, metal correlates to autumn, water correlates to winter, wood correlates to spring, and, as noted above, earth correlates to the "in between" seasons, when the energies are in transition, something we can probably understand most easily with the energies of late summer, as "Indian" summer. The vibrancy of the elements fluctuates throughout the year—water is stronger in the winter, fire is stronger in the summer months, and so on (see table 2.3).

In eating seasonally one addresses both the element and the environment involved. The current season plays a central role in which foods you may choose to eat. In the summer (the fire element, hot) we require more cooling foods, and in the winter (the water element, cold) we require more warming, deeply nourishing foods. When we are thinking of foods to enhance our elemental balance, we should also take into account the seasonality of the foods we consume.

TABLE 2.2. ELEMENTS, SEASONS, FLAVORS, COLORS, AND ORGANS

ELEMENT	SEASON	FLAVOR(S)/ TASTE(S)	COLOR(S)	YIN ORGAN(S)	YANG ORGAN
FIRE	Summer	Bitter	Red, purple, pink	Heart	Small intestine
EARTH	All "in between" seasons, such as "Indian" summer	Sweet	Yellow, beige, brown	Spleen, pancreas	Stomach
METAL	Autumn	Pungent, hot	White, gold, silver, bronze	Lungs	Large intestine
WATER	Winter	Salty	Black, dark blue	Kidneys	Bladder
WOOD	Spring	Sour	Green, light blue, turquoise	Liver	Gallbladder

TABLE 2.3. ELEMENTS AND THEIR SEASONS

ELEMENT	SEASONS	MONTHS	DATES
EARTH	In-between seasons	January, early February	1/6–2/3
WOOD	Spring	February, March, early April	2/4–4/4
EARTH	In-between seasons	April, early May	4/5–5/4
FIRE	Summer	May, June, early July	5/5–7/6
EARTH	In-between seasons	July, early August	7/7–8/6
METAL	Autumn	August, September, early October	8/7–10/7
EARTH	In-between seasons	October, early November	10/8–11/6
WATER	Winter	November, December, early January	11/7–1/5

THE FIVE FLAVORS, OR TASTES

Just as each element is characterized by a season, so too each has a correlative taste (see table 2.2 on page 37). Fire is bitter taste, earth is sweet taste, metal is pungent (or hot or spicy) taste, water is salty taste, and wood is sour taste. A food rarely is one of these tastes exclusively, although there is often a predominant taste. Also, just because flavor is generally associated with a particular element, this does not mean that *only* foods of predominantly that taste will be best for the nutritional balance of the organs of that element. In other words, in the table of foods to balance the fire organs (see the fire chapter) you will find foods of a variety of predominant flavors, not just bitter foods.

In addition to the element associations, each flavor supports a specific organ or organ system and is associated with a season. It is said that a little of a particular taste can strengthen an element or organ system, whereas an excess of it can impede proper function. Hence, too much sugar (sweet) plays havoc with your earth energy (stomach, spleen, pancreas) and contributes to digestive problems. As with everything, balance is key. Below is a summary of the flavors along with some examples of food sources.

Bitter: associated with early to midsummer and fire; stimulating to heart and small intestine; foods include dandelion (leaf and root), kale, parsley, and rye

Salty: associated with winter and water; strengthening to kidneys and bladder; foods include alfalfa sprouts, artichoke, sardine, and seaweed

Sweet: associated with very late summer ("Indian" summer) and earth; influences pancreas, spleen, and stomach; foods include apple, banana, beet, pumpkin, and sunflower seed (note that "sweet" does not equate to "sweets," as in foods artificially sweetened by sugar or other sweeteners)

Sour: associated with spring and wood; energizes liver and gallbladder; foods include adzuki bean, cranberry, blackberry, and lemon

Pungent: associated with autumn and metal; influences lungs and colon; foods include garlic, ginger, horseradish, onion, and sage

THE FIVE COLORS

As noted in the Inner Smile Meditation combined with the Healing Sounds exercise in chapter 1, there are also colors associated with each of the elements (see table 2.2 on page 37). Red, purple, and pink are fire colors; yellow, orange, beige, and brown are earth colors; white, gold, silver, and bronze are metal colors; black and dark blue are water colors; and green, light blue, and turquoise are wood colors.

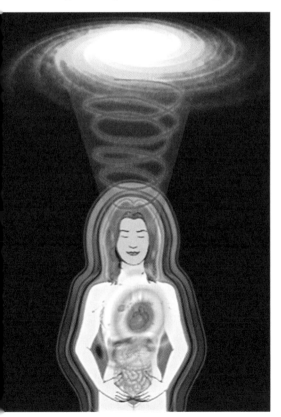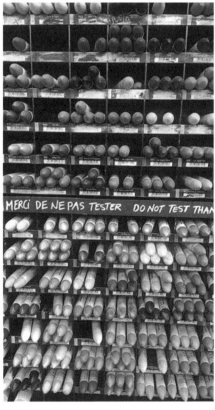

Fig. 2.4. It's a five-color world inside and out.

The most important principle in Taoist nutrition is to include all five elements in as many meals as possible through the five colors and five tastes while emphasizing your five-element remedy foods. Since many foods appear in more than one element list (included in each of the element chapters 4 through 8), you can follow your instincts with the five tastes and colors, mixing and matching according to your needs.

One easy way of adding all the five colors to your meal is by using garnishes. In the example of a spleen food like an omelette, you can add small pieces of black ingredients such as shiitake mushrooms (which are also called "black mushrooms"), along with some chopped tomato, some white onion to the omelette itself, and some parsley to garnish. Seaweeds have much nutritional value and come in several colors, as do onions and peppers. Bring out your inner five-color artist!

Taoists do not believe in one-food diets, where you eat only one thing to the exclusion of a varied diet. Upsetting the five-element balance in this way will always have negative consequences. Like the zoo mobile I hung above my baby son's cot, when he pulled on the giraffe,

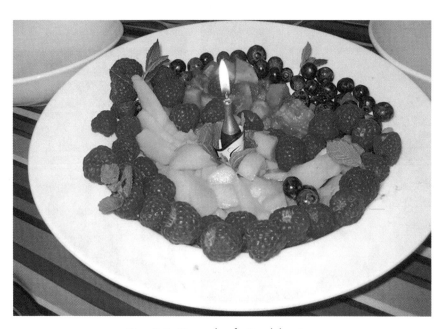

Fig. 2.5. Five-color fruit celebration

the elephant always went up in the air, the lion looked distressed, and the hippopotamus fell off. Traditional Chinese medicine always considers the effect on *all* the elements during a treatment; while the practitioner is looking for a remedy for a specific condition, he or she will also be treating possible side effects due to changing the balance of the elements. This is unlike the approach of Western allopathic medicine, which prescribes a pharmaceutical drug to treat a condition, but this will often mean that a second or third drug is needed to counteract all the side effects of the first one. So remember the interrelationship between all the elements when choosing your five-element nutrition.

ORGAN TIMING

You can optimize your digestion and the nutritional value of what you eat by enlisting the universe's prevailing twenty-four-hour energies. As the five elements' energies flow around the directions and seasons, they also flow around the hours of the day, influencing organ function at their prevailing high-energy time, like shining a spotlight on certain organs. Figs. 2.6 and 2.7 on pages 42 and 43 show visuals of the organ times and how they interact with our health and well-being.

The old adage, "Eat breakfast like a king, lunch like a prince, and dinner like a beggar" reflects the Taoist twenty-four-hour clock. Timing breakfast during the stomach time (7–9 a.m.) and spleen hours (9–11 a.m.) follows the peak digestion time of the large intestine (5–7 a.m.). This is also prime elimination time, so we can make room for the incoming food. After the good digestive hour we come into fire time and particularly the small intestine time between 1 p.m. and 3 p.m., so lunch at noon means there is further good digestion energy at this time. During the traditional Western tea or dinnertime, between, for example, 5 and 9 p.m. depending on the country, digestion energy is fairly low, which is why moderation at this meal is advised.

To properly use the prevailing energies during the twenty-four-hour cycle, we should ideally get up with the sun and go to bed when dark falls.

5 ELEMENT ORGANS		24 HOUR ORGAN TIME ZONE	RECOMMENDATIONS
FIRE	• Heart	11:00 a.m. – 1:00 p.m.	This is a good time to eat lunch; it is recommended to have a light, cooked meal.
	Absorption time		
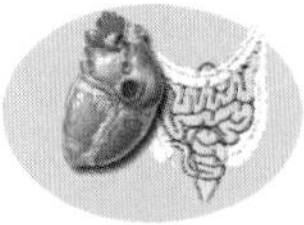	• Small Intestine	1:00 p.m. – 3:00 p.m.	This is a good time to go about daily tasks or exercise.
EARTH	• Stomach	7:00 a.m. – 9:00 a.m.	This is the time to eat the biggest meal of the day to optimize digestion and absorption.
	Digestion time		
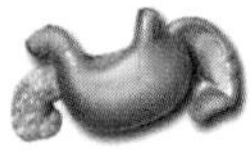	• Spleen — Pancreas	9:00 a.m. – 11:00 a.m.	Enzymes are released to help digest food and release energy for the day ahead. This is the ideal time to exercise and work.
METAL	• Lungs	3:00 a.m. – 5:00 a.m.	The lungs are at their peak energy in the early morning, you could schedule chi kung exercise at this time.
	Elimination time		
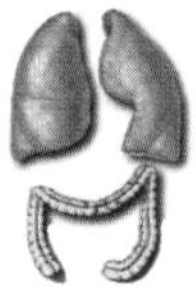	• Large Intestine	5:00 a.m. – 7:00 a.m.	Reserve enough time early in the morning for the large intestine's normal elimination function; this time is favorable for a bowel movement. It is also favorable for morning chi exercises.
WATER	• Bladder	3:00 p.m. – 5:00 p.m.	This is when metabolic wastes move into the kidney's filtration system. It is also a perfect time to study or complete brain-challenging work.
	Empty Elimination		
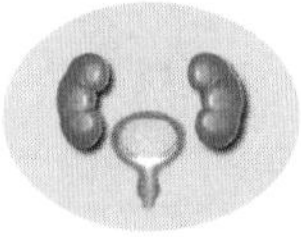	• Kidneys	5:00 p.m. – 7:00 p.m.	This is also the perfect time to study or complete brain-challenging work. Drinking a lot of water is advised to help aid detoxification.
WOOD	• Gallbladder	11:00 p.m. – 1:00 a.m.	The body should rest now in order to wake early in the morning feeling energized.
	Detoxification time		
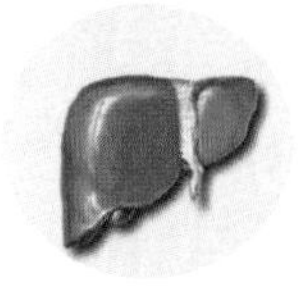	• Liver	1:00 a.m. – 3:00 a.m.	The liver cleanses the blood and performs a myriad of functions associated with daily activity, digestion, and elimination.

Fig. 2.6. Optimum daily structure according to organ timing

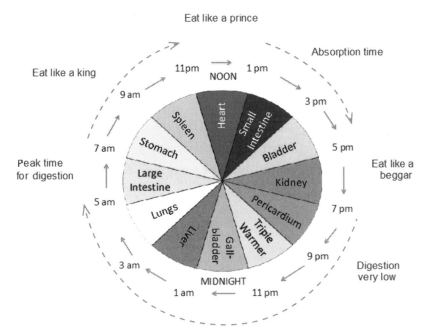

Fig. 2.7. Visual of meal timing according to organs and peak digestion.
(Note: The pericardium and triple warmer are important in Taoist
concepts of body functioning, in body work, and in meditations.
They fall under the fire element.)

Of course, the seasons affect the hours of sunrise and sunset, meaning
we sleep more in wintertime. From 11 p.m. to 3 a.m. our wood energies help the gallbladder and liver function properly, and during this
period the body should be at rest and not be taking in food to allow
this cleansing and detoxification work to happen efficiently. Should you
awaken in the middle of the night, it's good to drink some water in
order to help the flushing out of toxins, both from the liver work and
later from the large intestine (5–7 a.m.).

THE EFFECTS OF TEMPERATURE
AND COOKING

The study of human evolution is often marked by the point of "before
the discovery of fire" and after it. Once primitive humans discovered

fire, their brain, body, and indeed the entire species was now on a fast track to a different sort of development. Traditional Chinese cooking is mainly opposed to eating many vegetables and other foods raw, and the main concern is digestion. Today's nonprimitive humans do not spend most of their days hunting and eating wild foods. For primitive humans, a large part of their eating time involved many hours of masticating food in order to release its nutrients. Today, with an average eight-hour working day, our eating mode is vastly different from that of our early ancestors. Cooking food makes digestion a whole lot easier and allows us to accomplish many other activities. Cooking breaks down the connective tissue in meat and softens the cell walls in plants, allowing faster and better release of nutrients. A cooked portion of food can provide more energy than the same quantity raw. That's because cooking changes the chemical composition of food and also its chi. Take the example of an apple. Taoists considered it as overly cooling chi for the yin metal and yin fire organs (lungs and heart). However, its traditional Taoist nutritional qualities include many positives: stabilizing blood-sugar levels and body heat, neutralizing acidity, regulating the lungs, and preventing free-radical damage and inflammation, and its juice cleanses the gallbladder. So rather than avoiding apples, you could try lightly steaming or baking them; this will retain many of their best qualities while lessening their effects on cooling lung or heart chi should this be one of the things you need to be careful of in your five-element nutrition checklist.

The range of temperatures associated with the chi of a food are hot, warm, neutral, cool, and cold when applied to the yin and yang major organs associated with the five elements. If we want to strengthen the chi of an organ, we will choose foods that are hot or warm for that organ, as this means they will "heat" or stimulate the chi. We could also more easily avoid the foods that are cool or cold for that organ, to prevent further depletion of already low energy. If we have an organ that is overly strong and we wish to reduce it to harmonize the yin and yang and five elements, we would do the opposite. We would avoid the hot or warm foods associated with that organ, preferring the cold or cool ones.

As noted above, if a food you really want to eat is marked as cool and you wish to strengthen, you can move it into the warm column by cooking it. The cool food will not diminish chi as much when cooked. This allows us to not miss out on all the other benefits of cool foods, which have many qualities.

TAOIST SUPERFOODS

Many foods recommended in ancient Taoist lore on nutrition fit the modern definition of a superfood, a food that is especially rich in compounds such as antioxidants, fiber, or fatty acids, which are considered beneficial to a person's health by increasing energy and vitality, regulating cholesterol and blood pressure, and preventing cancer and other diseases. Foods such as the coconut have long been considered exceptional according to Taoist standards, while some foods are noteworthy for modern Western nutritional reasons. The East-meets-West delineation found here is by no means comprehensive, as an exhaustive study of modern superfoods is beyond the scope of this book. For more information on this subject there are numerous websites and a great deal of literature dealing with superfoods.

In fact, the information here only scratches the surface of what may be considered a Taoist superfood, as there are many other compounds that provide "super" nutrition other than the foods listed here. Traditional Chinese medicine possesses an incredibly deep well of knowledge for curing or correcting health conditions through foods that can be classified as superfoods according to the modern definition, and the information from TCM predates by far what modern Western medicine has to say about certain foods. For example, the coconut has recently been rehabilitated in the West, from being considered to contain unhealthy fat to being regarded as one of the very best superfoods around. Yet we should be wary of going overboard for any one food, even a superfood. Taoist nutrition advocates variety. The basic superfood information here is intended to help you with your food choices.

A few of the compounds that make a food a superfood include the following:

Antioxidants: These flush out harmful toxins from the body, thereby improving health and even resulting in a more streamlined body and glowing skin.

Beta-carotene: Yellow, red, and orange pigments characterize the carotenoid group; these natural chemical compounds are helpful in preventing eye conditions, cancer, Alzheimer's disease, blood pressure problems, and rheumatoid arthritis.

Beta-cryptoxanthin: Another carotenoid pigment, this strong antioxidant reduces the risk of arthritis and lung and colon cancers, as well as other cancers.

Beta-sitosterol: One of several plant sterols with a chemical structure similar to that of cholesterol, this substance lowers LDL "bad" cholesterol in the blood.

Ellagic acid: The antiproliferative and antioxidant properties of ellagic acid, a natural phenol antioxidant found in numerous fruits and vegetables, have prompted research into its potential health benefits, including its anticancer and antimutagenic properties.

Fiber: Fiber helps avoid constipation and hemorrhoids, as it facilitates transit through the digestive system.

Flavonoids: Flavonoids such as quercetin, kaempferol, catechins, and anthocyanins are ketone-containing compounds with antioxidant and anti-inflammatory properties that support the cardiovascular and nervous systems. They help detoxify and decrease the risk of some cancers.

Isothiocyanates: These are antioxidants and detoxifiers; cabbage, kale, broccoli, and cauliflower are some of the vegetables that have these natural substances, which have anticancer properties.

Low glycemic index: Glycemic index tells us how foods affect our blood sugar. Low glycemic-index foods are less likely to cause large or sudden increases in blood sugar levels; this is important in preventing or controlling diabetes, and also for weight management and prevention of cardiovascular disease. Many foods with a low glycemic index have a naturally sweet taste, so this cuts out the need to add sugar.

Lutein: A naturally occurring carotenoid, lutein, which is found in leafy green vegetables, such as mustard greens, has strong antioxidant effects.

Lycopene: A bright red carotene and phytochemical found in tomatoes and other red fruits and vegetables, lycopene is good for the blood and the heart, reduces risk of heart attack, and makes the skin look younger.

Zeaxanthin: A common carotenoid found in nature, in such foods as paprika, saffron, spirulina, and many dark green leafy vegetables, zeaxanthin is a potent antioxidant that helps protect the eyes from harmful rays and aging problems such as macular degeneration.

Each element also has specific superfoods that particularly support the organs associated with that element, and these can be found in each of the individual element chapters (chapters 4–8).

BASIC TAOIST PRINCIPLES OF EATING

Taoist philosophy emphasizes the way we eat and its relationship to our organs, our emotions, and the way we live. We must eat calmly and mindfully, thinking about what we eat and how we eat. The chi of food is a very important concept in Taoism—which is why we say locally grown and freshly harvested and freshly cooked food has the most chi. And chi in food is at the heart of five-element nutrition. The following guidelines are essential Taoist principles of eating:

Eat simply: The spleen governs our digestion, but too many ingredients do not necessarily combine well and make hard work for this organ. Simple food supports digestion better by not distressing the spleen. You can still respect this guideline while keeping the five colors and flavors rule in mind.

Eat light: Overeating congests the spleen and is a major cause of stagnation and dampness. Stop eating before you feel full, and set your mind to recognize when you feel two-thirds full. Otherwise the stomach will get used to being overstretched with too much food in it to break down—it can stretch to five times its own size and can lose its elasticity as a result. You will also lose much energy from the extra digestion needed to absorb too much food. Many traditional cultures express this idea of restraint when eating.

Reduce sugar: The spleen can become overwhelmed by too much sweet food, which causes intestinal fermentation that makes conditions ripe for parasites and yeast overgrowth; this further weakens the blood and depletes energy levels. Besides, the extra calories coming from sugar are rarely necessary.

Include naturally fermented foods: Include some naturally fermented foods in the diet such as sauerkraut, kimchi, or yogurt. The enzymes and probiotics contained in these kinds of foods can help digestion. Uncooked organic sauerkraut, either its juice or the solids in it, is considered very balancing, while in some regions of the world that are noted for longevity, people eat particular strains of natural plain yogurt.

Be mindful about food combining: Eat some foods separately from others; for example, fruit should not be eaten during the main meal. Fruits have a shorter digestion time, so eat them at least an hour before the main meal, and avoid eating them afterward as a dessert, as they will be stuck in a line behind slower-digesting foods and will start to ferment, producing painful gas. Cheese and meat take up to six hours to digest, and grains take two to four hours to digest, while fruit takes only two hours.

Salad greens have a short digestion time and should be eaten before the main dish, as indeed they often are eaten as a starter course. If they are tossed with some of the five flavors in a vinaigrette dressing, this will help to open the digestive flow. The principle of food combining will help support the spleen's function of sorting nutrients and will therefore reduce the possibility of digestive fermentation.

Limit drinking with meals: Too much fluid will dilute the essential digestive juices and overwhelm the spleen.

Avoid chilled food and iced drinks: Cold food slows down the digestive process because the digestive system must work harder to bring the temperature of nutrients up to match the stomach's temperature. Even in hot weather avoid drinking iced drinks and prefer hot teas instead, as receptors in the mouth will trigger a sweat response, which is cooling for the body. Chilled drinks do the opposite, canceling sweating and causing the blood vessels to constrict, which will keep you feeling hot in the long run. Cold beverages also impact the digestion, as digestive energy is wasted as the body attempts to regulate its core temperature. The Chinese believe that any fats or food eaten at the same time as a cold drink will become congealed, like oil solidifying in a fridge, impeding digestion and promoting stagnation in the intestines. As well, cold food and beverages make it harder for the spleen to work optimally, because this organ cannot function properly unless the body has sufficiently heated up the cold input. Cold food and beverages are also believed to produce mucus, making it difficult for asthmatics, while iced water can sometimes bring on headache.

Chew well: Chewing starts off the digestive process in the mouth, stimulating the body to preorder the digestive juices farther down. Also, well-chewed food demands less work for the stomach and intestines. If you chew each mouthful thirty times you will feel the saliva coming out, which is very important. In this way you can help predigestion as the saliva mixes with the food. If you add in air, although it is not always easy to eat with your mouth open in company, it makes the food still lighter and easier to digest.

Take your time eating: Activate the thyroid gland by eating more slowly and taking time to swallow. You can even very lightly massage your thyroid gland on your throat to aid this. The thyroid is like a spark plug—its function in digestion is to create more energy by assisting the reaction between the air ingested and the digestive process. The thyroid is located in a sensitive region of the body, in the throat—in fact kung fu blows there can be very dangerous. The modern style of eating fast means that digestion will actually take more energy, as we aren't giving the body a chance to work properly. The Tao talks about this: it is not just what you eat but what the body can absorb and make use of. As discussed in chapter 1, a relaxed vagus nerve is extremely important for maintaining the digestive system at its optimum, so slow eating along with the Inner Smile (see instructions in chapter 1, page 21) will help ensure proper digestion.

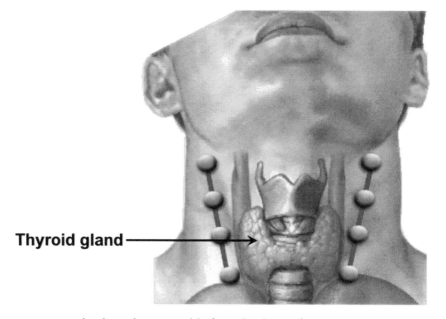

Thyroid gland

Fig. 2.8. The thyroid is accessible from the throat, for a gentle massage. Activate the thyroid gland further by eating slowly.

Eat when calm: Avoid eating in a hurry or when you feel worried, angry, or fearful. Try to have a rule not to talk about stressful things or watch TV at the dinner table so as not to agitate the emotions, which can adversely affect the vagus nerve and therefore the entire digestive system and the organs themselves. Keep in mind the five-element emotions.

Cook with love: Plan, prepare, and cook your meals with a loving heart. Appreciation for the food will be greater and digestion easier when this essential ingredient is included in each meal.

Cut vegetables according to how you cook them: Cut your vegetables according to the lines of the vegetable; for example, on a cucumber there are length-long lines, so it is better to cut this way, but of course in short strips rather than one cucumber length strip. The same goes for zucchini or other vegetables where you can see lines. How you cook vegetables is determined by their size and shape: larger pieces are for steaming, and thinner strips are for stir-fries. Combine flavors and colors for effect and taste, and cooking certain combinations of vegetables will bring out their flavor; get inspiration from a colorful South Asian cookbook!

Cooking methods: If you use charcoal to cook, you will have juicier food; gas is neutral, and electricity has a drying effect. Steaming food keeps in more nutrients, and you can also increase nutrient value by using the liquid from the steaming pan for sauces and soups or as a drink. Stir-frying also keeps in more nutrients. Cook by time and also smell to determine progress. The Chinese use light oil for stir-fries: safflower, sesame. Olive oil is too heavy for stir-fries but good on raw food and salads.

Eat food with the most chi: There are a few important rules to follow to ensure that the food you eat has the vital energy you need: Eat food grown locally that has not been transported a long distance. Prefer fresh food that has ripened on the tree or plant rather than harvested well before it has ripened to cut out "spoilage" during long transport. Eat freshly harvested food in season. Bear in mind that when food is harvested, brought to a store where it is purchased, and then stored in the fridge, it will already have less chi—which is why shopping at a local produce farmer's market is a good option. Avoid canned and preserved food, which is low in chi (such as delicious ham, which nevertheless is wanting in chi). Observe Hippocrates' dictum, "Let food be thy medicine and medicine be thy food."

There are a few other natural rules to observe when eating for optimum chi:

- Never add sugar or salt to baby food. When introducing real foods to a baby, let these be just pure fruits and vegetables. Babies will sometimes reject a food at first taste, as the taste is new to them. They might need to be offered the food several times before they will accept it; one theory says try it up to fifteen times before baby gets used to it, as they are in the process of educating their five flavors and deciding they like it, so don't give up on broccoli for your baby too quickly. Babies start off by accepting sweet things easily, and make sure these are naturally sweet foods, without any added sugar. The sweetness of breast milk is their first taste, and they are not generally ready for the other four tastes for several months (the exact timing is debated and depends on customs and foods commonly eaten in the family). Peel fruit and vegetables for young children, as the skins are usually a different taste and harder to digest. And avoid brown rice for the very young and very old as it is more of a challenge for an immature or sensitive digestive tract.
- Calcium can come in the form of bone broth, other kinds of meat stock (chicken broth, beef broth), leafy green vegetables, and seaweeds. These are all fine for anyone, and for babies once they've been weaned. Milk and dairy products are often pro-

moted for their calcium content, but other calcium-rich foods such as leafy green vegetables and grasses are a good substitute for dairy. Remember, cows become big creatures with huge bones by eating grasses.

Eating too many acidic foods such as meat can result in a situation where the body takes calcium from the bones to help neutralize the overly acidic condition caused from eating so many animal products. This is actually a calcium-robbing situation rather than a calcium-deficiency problem. As long as you eat an alkalizing diet that is rich in green foods and drinks, you don't need to worry about getting adequate calcium.

- When the body receives a lot of high-calorie food and fats, it goes into panic mode. It will take those calories and store the extra fat in fat cells, but then it is as if it forgets where it has put it. So those unhealthy fats are stockpiled, and they become difficult to access for energy and difficult to shake off if you want to redefine your figure. The more calories you eat, the more your body will store. And when stored in the form of fat deposits that the body cannot access instantaneously, a process must happen before this fat can be put to use. One such process is fasting, but when you fast at one level the body panics even more, so when you finish the fast, you eat to excess, starting the cycle all over again and causing the weight to return.* The solution, of course, is to follow the guidelines for nutrition outlined in this book. When the organs are happy and the emotions are good, then the body will be happy and will function better. And if you are sometimes forced to eat irregularly, make sure you eat a good meal, slowly, and that all the five elements and their organs are happy.

- Be careful with fungus foods. Mushrooms, truffles, and algae are all acid-forming foods that contain mycotoxins, a product of

---

*If you are interested in fasting, read *Pi Gu Chi Kung: Inner Alchemy Energy Fasting,* by Mantak Chia and Christine Harkness-Giles, on the ancient energizing fast.

yeast that poisons the body's tissues and cells. The mushroom is not really a vegetable but rather the fruiting body of a yeast or fungus. Yeast is to be avoided (as are yeast-containing alcoholic beverages). Many mushrooms are poisonous; however, some are considered to have longevity and health-giving virtues such as shiitake (also called "black mushrooms") and are eaten for such benefits. Note that mushrooms are acid, so if you want to eat them, add them to alkaline vegetables to neutralize the acidity. In fact, in China mushrooms are not generally eaten on their own. Gout and rheumatism are conditions that are worsened with acid; therefore, avoid yeasts and mushrooms if you suffer from these conditions. However, eating a lemon a day helps neutralize these kinds of acid-forming foods, as lemon is actually an alkaline-forming fruit, even though it has an acid taste. Therefore lemon is often recommended for these conditions.

- Avoid tobacco completely—either smoking or chewing it. In addition to the well-known dangers of tobacco the leaves are also coated with mycotoxin due to fermentation. This is another reason tobacco is poisonous to the body.

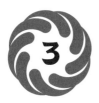

Applying Five-Element Nutrition Using Inner Alchemy Astrology

To use the theory of five-element nutrition for healing, for optimum health, or to maintain well-being, you must begin with your unique five-element profile. That profile will provide some clues as to why siblings in the same family, eating the same foods, having the same DNA will have different bodies, attitudes, virtues, and difficulties. Nature, nurture, and especially one's own natal astrology—the five elemental energies we are each born with—all point to an explanation of why this is so.

The importance of each of the five elements is equal, and they are interdependent. They have an influence over your life and the major organs in your body. They arc forces or energies in the cosmos. "As above, so below." The five energies are not only in the cosmos, they are also in your body. Your astrological chart for the time you were born will reveal which of your five elements are out of balance, although you will have probably already noticed the effects of any imbalances in terms of your emotional tendencies and physical problems. It is helpful to know that you can harmonize your elements and balance your energies with correct five-element nutrition, Taoist practices, and a healthy lifestyle.

There is an old Taoist adage that goes like this: "The five organs are like five children—you have to satisfy them with the five emotions, the five colors, the five smells, and the five tastes." Applying these basics, we keep the body happy and balanced with the Inner Smile and Healing Sounds meditation (described in chapter 1, page 21), smiling in positive virtues and clearing out negative emotions. We also make sure the five colors and five tastes are represented on our plate when we eat. This very age-old wisdom from Taoist sages will make for a happy and healthy life.

DETERMINING YOUR OWN FIVE-ELEMENT MAKEUP

In the previous chapters we looked at how we classify foods according to the five elements to harmonize and balance the prevailing energies of the major organs, which are each associated with one of the five elements. Now we will consider how five-element nutrition can be applied to your unique element profile as determined by your astrological makeup. You don't need to be an expert in Chinese astrology or to do complex calculations to ascertain your basic Inner Alchemy astrological makeup. This can be easily and quickly calculated by inputting your birth data at Master Chia's website, **https://www.universal-tao.com /InnerAlchemyAstrology**. Your Inner Alchemy astrology will calculate your unique five-element makeup at the time of your birth, giving you insight into the balance of your organs, emotions, sense organs, and types of actions in your life on the level of chi, or vital energy.

The online calculation will give you your natal chart table, or Bazi chart, on the left-hand side of the webpage, and from that a calculation of your energies is made into a pictogram of the five elements using their colors, on the right-hand side (see fig. 3.1 on page 58 for an example). In the pictogram, each element bubble will show a percentage of the element, indicating the strength or weakness of that element in your personal makeup. Note that 20 percent is the mean, so we would consider roughly 16 to 24 percent to be "normal." More than this would represent an excess and less a deficiency. But as you will see below, according to the creating cycle of the elements, the element itself could also be generously or poorly supported by the element preceding it. By examining the interaction of the elements in your chart, you can easily learn how to support any imbalances. This can be done either by feeding a weak element or by draining an overly strong element. It is particularly important to focus on your day master as determined by your chart—boosting a weak day master and cutting down a strong one.

Day Master and Organ Strength

The day master is the all-important starting point for interpreting an authentic Chinese astrology chart because this is the element that represents *you*. While the Chinese year animal has some relevant characteristics and is better known, it is the day master that provides much deeper information about a person's energies, talents, emotions, five-element nutrition, and relationship to all areas of life.

You can determine your day master in your Inner Alchemy astrology personal chart by looking at the top two lines in the "day" column of the natal chart. For example, in fig. 3.1, on page 58, the day master is yin metal. Your day master refers to the day on which you were born, or more specifically the dominant chi on the day of your birth. It is the element that most represents your "self" in either a yin or yang polarity of that element. There are ten possible day masters, a yin and yang version of each of the five elements. So be aware of your day master polarity.

However, if this day master element occurs more than once in the natal table on the left, then look at how many yin and how many yang appearances there are of that element. This will also talk about your organs and the strength of the organ energies. Chapter 1 discussed the

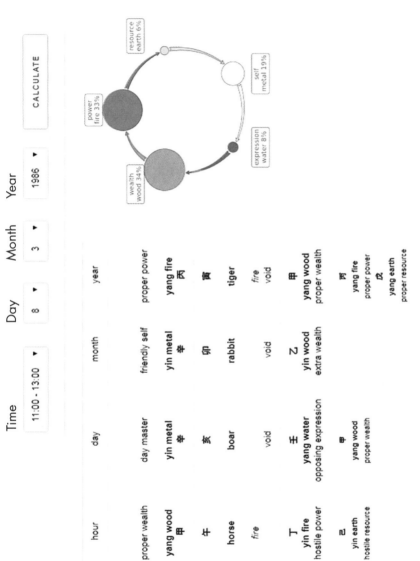

Fig. 3.1. Screenshot of a sample Universal Tao Inner Alchemy astrology birth chart. Across the top is where the birth data is entered; on the left is the natal chart, and on the right is the element pictogram.

yin and yang organ pairs, and you can find them in table 1.1 (page 17). In the example in fig. 3.1, the day master is yin metal, and in the natal chart this appears twice with no yang metal appearing, which indicates that the yin metal organ, the lungs, is stable, but the yang organ, the large intestine, may need more support. Note also that the percentage of metal (day master/self) in the pictogram is 19 percent, falling within the "normal" or balanced range. In another example, if you are yin metal and your day master/self is fairly weak, it would be important to give the yin metal organ extra support in terms of food consumed with possibly less focus on the yang organ if that were more abundant.

You can continue these observations with the other four elements, using the same method of counting the yin and yang appearances in the natal table on the left of your chart.* Using the example of fig. 3.1, table 3.1 on page 60 shows a full organ analysis based on this natal chart. You can create your own version of this table based on your chart by filling in the values in a blank table, such as table 3.2 on page 60. Note that 0 indicates deficient energy, 1 and 2 indicate balanced energy, and 3 (or more) indicate high or excess energy. So our example chart indicates deficient energy in the large intestine and kidneys, excessive energy in the gallbladder, and balanced energy in the other organs.

Below are general descriptions of the personality traits of the ten day masters. The strength of your day master (shown by the percentage in your pictogram) together with the quantity and quality of the other four elements in your natal chart will affect how much the description and traits of your day master apply to you. Using this information in combination with the familial and phase relationships between the elements described below, you can better understand how to support your day master nutritionally and otherwise by balancing the other elements

---

*If you would like a much deeper view, the "full chart" for purchase on the Universal Tao Inner Alchemy website will do that for you. But there is already much useful information for you in the natal or Bazi chart.

TABLE 3.1. ORGAN ANALYSIS FOR SAMPLE CHART (FIG. 3.1)

ELEMENT	ORGAN	VALUE
Yin Fire	Heart	1
Yang Fire	Small intestine	2
Yin Earth	Spleen, pancreas	1
Yang Earth	Stomach	1
Yin Metal	Lungs	2
Yang Metal	Large intestine	0
Yin Water	Kidneys	0
Yang Water	Bladder	1
Yin Wood	Liver	1
Yang Wood	Gallbladder	3

TABLE 3.2. YOUR ORGAN ANALYSIS CHART

Fill in the Blank Values to Determine Your Organ Strength

ELEMENT	ORGAN	VALUE
Yin Fire	Heart	
Yang Fire	Small intestine	
Yin Earth	Spleen, pancreas	
Yang Earth	Stomach	
Yin Metal	Lungs	
Yang Metal	Large intestine	
Yin Water	Kidneys	
Yang Water	Bladder	
Yin Wood	Liver	
Yang Wood	Gallbladder	

and aspects of your life. The self-awareness that comes from examining your day master can also help you understand your relationship to food and how the physical, emotional, mental, and spiritual aspects of our being *all* contribute to our overall health and well-being.

Yang fire day master: Yang fire is like the sun—it radiates warmth and light, and these day masters can be generous, open, sincere, just, upright, noble, vibrant, explosive, passionate, independent, and outgoing. They can also be selfish, lonely, arrogant, opinionated, relentless, and bossy and can sometimes think the world revolves around them. Born leaders and warriors, yang fire day masters are good talkers but not always good listeners.

Yin fire day master: Yin fire is glowing moonlight and candles; it is mild, gentle, adventurous, diplomatic, private, conservative, courteous, warm, deep, careful, cautious, and unhurried and pays attention to detail. Yin fire day masters are sentimental, inspirational, and motivating. They can be good friends—sensitive and tolerant. They are fast thinkers, taking pride in leading and illuminating others and in careful planning. They can also be fickle and do not always communicate their feelings or their plans and actions, which tends to irritate others.

Yang earth day master: Yang earth is like a high mountain or a deep canyon. These day masters can be very protective and can be counted on as loyal friends. They are trustworthy, caring, dependable, optimistic, and solid, with their feet on the ground. They can also be stubborn, inflexible, immovable, and willful. Their consistency and sense of justice is inspiring to others, and they have good social and organizational skills; however, their inflexibility and chronic worrying can compromise their projects.

Yin earth day master: Yin earth is the moist soil from field and garden; if this earth is wet it can easily be washed away in the rains. Yin earth day masters have a high level of understanding and learning; their grasp of knowledge is rapid, and they are intellectually versatile, with a soft, flexible, comfortable nature. They inspire confidence to handle difficult problems. Good at managing people, they are tolerant, resourceful, and creative, as well as good-hearted and dependable, and they are driven to improve themselves. They can lack adaptability and have a hard time making quick, spontaneous decisions. Worry can disable their projects and concentration levels, and sometimes they are taken for granted by others.

Yang metal day master: Yang metal is the strong and powerful metal that can be made into swords or other weapons. These day masters are tough, driven, selfless, righteous, direct, sharp, tenacious, and determined and do not like to admit to failure. Yang metal has endurance and stamina and can tolerate hardship and suffering to achieve goals, with hands-on methods. They know how to build a team, communicate, and analyze a situation. They can lack flexibility and can be hasty in action, not paying attention to the finer details. They show enthusiasm and determination in whatever they do, but they may not always express their inner feelings. They can be cutting in their remarks to others, making enemies easily.

Yin metal day master: Yin metal is gold and the fine metals of jewelry. These day masters are beautiful, gentle, sensitive, attention seeking, sentimental, easily approachable, helpful, and expressive. They have fine feelings, unique opinions, and big hearts and are generous. They want the best. They make good friends, but they are often on show and seek the limelight. They love the new, the beautiful, the latest, so they can seem vain. They can also be opinionated, sharp, driven, and interested in appearances. They are good with money and make good bankers and decision makers, and they have relentless energy for work and projects.

Yang water day master: Yang water is the ocean, lake, river, or turbulent water. Yang water day masters are intelligent, clean, adaptable, gentle, softhearted, enthusiastic, likable, extroverted, rebellious, good communicators, determined, resourceful, and always on the move, sometimes with violent energy. They love adventure and physical activity; they flow around obstacles, neglect comforts, and show little sign of worry as they surf toward their goal. Their fluidity can lead to many distractions from the task at hand, as they can lose focus on their objectives. Fear can let them down.

Yin water day master: Yin water is a soft, gentle moisture like dew. These day masters are peaceful, diligent, hardworking, imaginative, adaptable, steady, calm, philosophical, likable, creative, and good teachers or communicators. Yin water day masters do not sit still for long. They can be cool, clearheaded, and sensitive to others' feelings but don't manage their own feelings well, tending to keep things private. They commonly harbor fantasies and romantic thoughts. They value principles and can see the greater good. They are led by their hearts when pursuing careers or dreams.

Yang wood day master: Yang wood is the energy of a large tree: strong, powerful, steady, forthright, direct, stern, down-to-earth, straightforward, sturdy, stubborn, unbending, reliable, supportive, outspoken, determined, righteous, deep-rooted, and serious. Yang wood day masters have strong willpower and don't give up easily in the face of adversity. Their reputation and morals are important to them. They are sympathetic to those in need of help but can also be authoritarian, bossy, predictable, slow-witted, and slow to change or compromise. They can be thick skinned when it comes to understanding what is happening around them, giving the impression that they are uncaring.

Yin wood day master: Yin wood is vegetation such as flowers and plants—soft and mild, but also flexible, adaptable, expressive, extroverted, charismatic, creative, quick-witted, possessive, careful, and good with money. Yin wood day masters are survivors, good motivators, and good project leaders. They know how to skirt around trouble but can also be timid and easily swayed and can change their mind and strategy easily according to circumstances. With a tendency to hold grudges, they may be easily deceived, but if well rooted they can survive a storm easier than yang wood.

THE CYCLES OF THE ELEMENTS

As we know, the five elements interact with one another. In your chart that interaction is shown in a cycle of five circles, as shown in fig. 3.2.

Additionally there are four important cycles that describe the interrelationships between the five elements and how they either support or weaken one another. These interrelationships are often explained using the metaphor of the family constellation. These four are:

Generating cycle: This goes clockwise in the direction fire, earth, metal, water, wood, fire, earth, and so on, as shown by the "generating" arrows in fig. 3.3. Each element "feeds" the next one, such that fire feeds earth, earth feeds metal, metal feeds water, and so on, as the pattern continues ad infinitum. Thus the "parent" element feeds the "child" element, making the element that follows in this clockwise direction the child.

Weakening cycle: This is the generating cycle in reverse, in which the elements go in the opposite, counterclockwise, direction—fire, wood, water, metal, earth, fire, wood, and so on, as shown by the "weakening" arrows in fig. 3.3. The feeding element is weakened by the feeding it is doing: fire weakens wood, wood weakens water, water weakens metal, and so forth. In other words, the parent element is weakened by giving to the next element, in the same way that it takes energy for a mother to feed her baby or for parents to give their energy to their children.

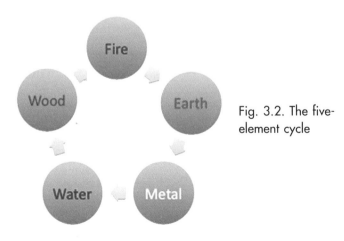

Fig. 3.2. The five-element cycle

Controlling cycle: Each element controls the element two away from it (the element after the child, moving clockwise) and is in turn controlled by the element that comes two before (the element before the parent, moving counterclockwise). So fire controls metal, metal controls wood, wood controls earth, earth controls water, water controls fire. Note that fire melts metal when it controls it, just as metal cuts wood, wood imprisons earth, earth dries up water, and water extinguishes fire as shown by the "controlling" arrows in fig. 3.3. Using the

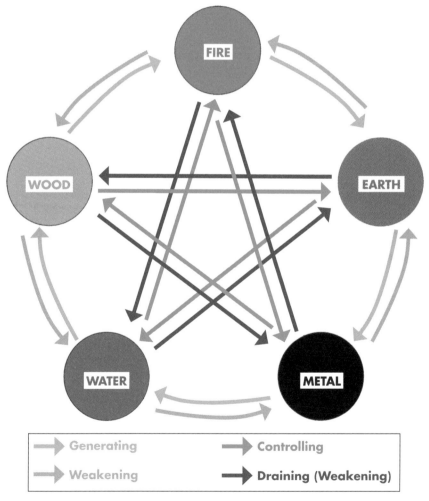

Fig. 3.3. Interrelationship of elements as shown through the supporting and weakening cycles

family metaphor, we say the controller is the "grandparent" and the element controlled is the "grandchild." For example, in the fire-controls-metal relationship, fire is the grandparent and metal is the grandchild. Fire's grandparent is therefore water.

Draining (or Weakening) Cycle: The controlling cycle in reverse gives another weakening cycle inasmuch as holding on to control is tiring, as shown by the "draining" arrows in fig. 3.3. When an element is controlling another one, it is effectively weakened, but the sizes of the elements decide how weakening this would be. In other words, the grandchild is both controlled by and weakening to the grandparent. Ancient Chinese texts on astrology talked about "insulting" as the opposite reaction to control, a sort of antagonism.

These four cycles are expressed as a family constellation in Taoist astrology, as shown in the table 3.3.

TABLE 3.3. FAMILY AND PHASE* OF ELEMENTS

ELEMENT	SIBLING / SELF	PARENT / RESOURCE	CHILD / EXPRESSION	GRANDCHILD / WEALTH	GRANDPARENT / POWER
FIRE	Fire	Wood	Earth	Metal	Water
EARTH	Earth	Fire	Metal	Water	Wood
METAL	Metal	Earth	Water	Wood	Fire
WATER	Water	Metal	Wood	Fire	Earth
WOOD	Wood	Water	Fire	Earth	Metal

*Note that the phase is indicated in the pictogram on your natal chart.

To summarize, the grandparent is considered the controller and the grandchild the one controlled or draining, another form of weakening. Please note that the Inner Alchemy practices are about nourishing the elements and having good chi flow around the five elements within us, rather than attacking one element with another. The Inner Smile Meditation (see page 21) is a good example of this, with each organ/element feeding the next one as we generate energy through smiling at our organs inside of ourselves. In this way the chi flows through our organs, and the five elements, in the direction of the creating cycle, and promotes harmony and balance.

The parent is the generating source, feeding the element in question, and the child weakens the parent. The sibling is the same as the self, the element in question, therefore supporting it. This also represents your peers, colleagues, people who share an interest with you, and people of your generation. You can apply this family relationship to your own Inner Alchemy astrological makeup using the pictogram on your chart in the same way—starting with the element identified as "self" (which is also your day master). The first element after it, moving clockwise, is your child, the first element directly before it, moving counterclockwise, is your parent, and so on. You will also notice that the column headings in table 3.3 identify the "phase" related to each of these familial relationships, beginning with the self phase we have already mentioned. These five phases are also important in understanding our five-element makeup and how to balance it.

THE FIVE PHASES

The role of each element in your life is determined by its relationship to the day master. In addition to the familial relationship, there are also the five phases, or actions in your life. The quantity of these five phases in your chart and the relationships between them also contribute to your level of chi, or vital energy. These five phases, or actions, are *self, expression, wealth, power, and resource.* Each of the five phases is calculated for you on one of the bubbles in the pictogram and is of that element energy in your individual makeup. Each of these also has a yin and a yang aspect, making a total of ten phases, known in Chinese astrology as *ten gods.* These yin or yang polarities for your own phases can be found in your basic chart calculations in the natal chart on the left by locating the yin or yang elements noted as "proper" expression, wealth, and so on (see the sample chart in fig. 3.1, page 58).

Regardless of whether or not you know the main polarity of your phases, it is important to balance the phases in your life nutritionally and otherwise. Chinese astrology advice is based on the basic premise of whether the day master is weak or strong. A rough guide will be to add together the percentages of your self and your resource phases. This is your "team," and the other three phases are then considered the "other team," by which you are drained every day. Excesses in either direction will give us a weak or strong day master. Looking for balance we will support and feed a weak day master to have energy to continue daily tasks and weaken a strong day master to spread out that chi around the five element cycle to make the other phases higher performing. Just as when working out we would not try to strengthen just one set of muscles, we would not seek to give a strong day master mainly its element food.

Self is the day master; it represents you, and it also describes your peers, friends, and competitors, people of the same energy as you. For instance, if you are wood, then wood people are your peers. Your self can denote your self-esteem and confidence and also ambitions and purpose. So Chinese astrology refers to a "weak day master" or a "strong day master" when making calculations. However, these don't always correlate in ways you might assume. For instance, a large quantity of this day master element in your chart does not necessarily mean you will have a lot of friends, because a strong day master can be very opinionated and not get along well with other people, whereas a weak day master might be more open to listening to other energies and could therefore potentially have more friends. The other phases should be compared in strength to your day master as noted by their size and percentage in the pictogram. This is very important when interpreting a chart.

Expression is your child, project, work, action, assertions, and your showing your true feelings. It represents our intelligence and ability and can indicate motivation in regard to work represented by that element's energy. You nourish and give birth to this element, but all of that nurturing can weaken you if this element is much stronger than your self element. Being low in expression could mean difficulty in showing your true self and asserting yourself. Being high in expression could mean that you're always on the go; you don't go in for relaxation and might not sleep much, all this is draining for a day master. The presence of this expression phase is a powerful antidote to the absence of other elements. When there is also a good wealth element, or wealth coming into the chart, then this expression element helps you to take advantage of the wealth being offered. It is your work, and without working you cannot hope to cash in on prosperity available in your wealth phase.

Wealth is what the day master controls, the grandchild, but the day master can also be drained or weakened by this element, by the obligation to control it, if it is overly strong. Although Western society can be coy about personal interest in money, to Chinese society it is seen as a form of energy with no shame attached to desiring it. So wealth, or prosperity, accompanied by good health and a long life, is considered most fortunate. It implies success and achievement but needs some expression phase to realize its potential.

Power is the element that controls us, the grandparent. It can give you structure and self-discipline. Too much of this element can be overpowering for your day master, but controlling is tiring, and you can also wear this element out. A balanced amount of this element is essential to grasp the organizational skills necessary to achieve what you want or need to do.

Resource is the energy that nourishes you, gives you ideas, and supports you—the parent element. Knowledge and thinking stem from this element. Too much resource can be suffocating or overwhelming or even leave you lazy. Not enough can create feelings of insecurity or feeling that you lack a support system—familial or otherwise. On a more positive note, weak resource could generate a desire to constantly learn new things and broaden education to fill this void.

We can see how the family cycles and phases work together with the example of the first line in table 3.3 where the day master/self is described by the element water, and its sibling is water, the same element, like a brother, sister, or peer. Its parent and resource is metal—metal feeds it. Water's child and expression is wood, as water feeds wood, which is also depleting to water. Its grandchild and wealth is fire, as water controls fire, but fire could also have the weakening potential to evaporate water if the quantity is larger than the water's. And its grandparent and power is earth, as earth controls water, but water could have the weakening potential to erode earth—if there are not enough sandbags, then the flood water will get in.

When looking at these phases in terms of nutrition, you need to support your own energy, your self, before supporting those around you—your family—and successfully dealing with the things you have to do in life—your other phases.

HOW TO APPLY FIVE-ELEMENT NUTRITION TO YOUR BIRTH CHART

Now that you better understand Taoist nutrition and Inner Alchemy astrology, it's time to put the two together to see how you can apply them to your own birth chart to make balanced nutritional choices.

Applying Nutrition to Your Day Master

As explained earlier in the chapter, your day master is you; it describes your underlying energies, character, and emotional framework and is shown as *self* on the pictogram, so begin by examining and balancing your day master. Your chart will show you whether your day master and its accompanying organs are weak or strong in terms of the percentage in your pictogram and the number of yin and yang appearances of your day master in the natal chart. You can use your resource element to help nourish your self element and achieve more balance there. If your day master is weak, you will want to support it with foods from your day master's element food list and that of the resource element. If it is overly strong, you may want to cut back on some of these foods.

But you have also learned more complex ways to support your day master by looking at it in comparison to your other elements, relationships, and phases. You may want to print out your astrological chart and write in the family relationships so that you can get a better sense of your own generating and weakening cycles. And you can also create your own table of relationships, as in table 3.4, to create a different visual for yourself.

TABLE 3.4. YOUR ELEMENTAL RELATIONSHIPS AND PHASES

Fill in the Blank Spaces Based on Your Natal Chart

ELEMENT	RELATIONSHIP	PHASE	PERCENTAGE
Day Master:	Self/Sibling	Self	
	Child	Expression	
	Grandchild	Wealth	
	Grandparent	Power	
	Parent	Resource	

In table 3.4 you would fill in the first column with your elements, starting with your self element and moving clockwise, and the last column with your corresponding percentages. Then, looking at both your table and pictogram, you could note which elements are weakening to your day master—child, grandchild, and sometimes even grandparent—and which are supporting or generating—parent and sometimes grandparent. If your weakening elements (the expression, wealth, and power phases) are overly strong, you may want to avoid foods that strengthen those elements further. If your supporting elements are quite weak (self and resource phases), you may want to bolster your day master by eating foods from those element lists. However, remember that balance is key to nutrition, and that the balance within our other elements also factors into our overall well-being.

Balancing Your Other Elements

You have learned above that *more* is not necessarily *better,* so we want to make sure we look at our elemental profile as a whole. Remember from the discussion above, for instance, that a parent who provides *too much* support (a high percentage) could create laziness or lack of ambition, while an unsupportive parent has the potential to breed self-motivation as a positive side effect. So beyond looking at your day master and its relationship to the other elements, you also want to take into account each phase or action in your chart.

In addition to looking at how these phases factor into your birth chart, into your life as a whole, you also want to acknowledge your own intuition of how these elements and phases are interacting with your life as it is now. Our birth chart shows our overall makeup, but our lives are composed of many phases and cycles. You can get more information about and precise readings of these phases and cycles of life by purchasing a more in-depth Inner Alchemy astrology chart or getting an Inner Alchemy astrology reading from a Universal Healing Tao Life Energy reader or astrologer (more on this in The Influence of Incoming Energies, page 86). You can also use your own observations based on what we've learned so far to get a sense of where balance is needed in your life and consider how this fits in with your life as experienced up to now.

Take a moment to review the descriptions of the four cycles on pages 64 to 67 and five phases on pages 67 to 70 as well as your own elements and percentages for those phases. Also review the organ analysis table you created as well as the descriptions of the organs and their corresponding emotions in chapter 1. Try sitting quietly five or ten minutes to bring awareness to the balance (or imbalance) of these relationships, actions, emotions, and elements in your own life.

Use the knowledge of your chart, your self-awareness, and the Taoist principles of nutrition introduced in the first two chapters to determine the best food choices to balance your elements and your life based on the food tables in the individual element chapters that follow. Remember that balance is key.

READING THE FOOD TABLES

Now that you have a better understanding of your own element profile you can begin to use nutrition as a tool to create more balance in your body and your life. Each of the element chapters that follow contain tables of foods that nurture or affect that element and the related organs. These tables can also all be found in the appendices at the back of the book for easy reference as you are creating your balanced nutrition plan. Table 3.5 below is a sample from the earth foods table.

TABLE 3.5. SAMPLE OF FOODS THAT SUPPORT EARTH ORGANS AND HEALTH

FOOD	FLAVOR(S)	TEMPERATURE	YIN ORGANS	YANG ORGAN
Alfalfa seed	Bitter	Cool	Spleen, pancreas	Stomach
Alfalfa sprout	Salty, bitter	Cool	Spleen, pancreas	Stomach
Aloe vera	Bitter	Neutral	Spleen, pancreas	Stomach
Apricot	Sweet, sour	Neutral	Spleen, pancreas	
Avocado	Sweet	Cool	Spleen, pancreas	

The tables include the important Taoist nutrition information of the flavor (or taste) and temperature of the foods, as well as which of the element's organs the food helps support. Remember that cool or cold brings down the chi of the organ(s) indicated and that each flavor is also associated with an element, so looking at flavors may be another way to bolster a weak element or organ in your chart. Also note that there is crossover between the food tables—certain foods appear in more than one table, and each table contains foods of a variety of flavors and colors.

Based on the information we've learned in these first three chapters, here is a recap of how the food tables might be used:

1. Review your natal chart and pictogram, and create your own versions of the organ analysis and elemental relationship and phases tables (table 3.2 on page 60 and table 3.4 on page 71).

2. Decide from these tables which elements are out of balance and which of the "ten gods"—yin fire, yang fire, yin earth, and so on—is deficient or excessive. Remember that in the organ analysis 0 indicates deficient energy, 1 and 2 indicate balanced energy, and 3 (or more) indicate high or excess energy.

3. See which organs—continuing from the examples in step 2: heart, small intestine, spleen and pancreas, and so on—need energetic improvement, starting with the most imbalanced first, the zeros or excessive highs. Pay particular attention to your day master organs.

4. Look at the food table for the element that corresponds to that organ as well as the food tables for the specific organ itself, and note which foods apply, keeping in mind that cool and cold foods will decrease chi, or energy, and warm or hot foods will increase it. In other words, if we have a deficiency we are going to avoid cool or cold foods for that organ and for an excess we are going to avoid hot or warm foods for that organ.

5. See how you can incorporate those foods into your diet.

Remembering to avoid certain foods is sometimes easier than deciding to bring different foods into your diet. If there are several different organs/elements to be supported, check the impact of your choices for one organ on the other organs that need support. That is why a good starting point is the organ energy that is most imbalanced.

SAMPLE READINGS

The following are sample readings of some well-known figures to give you a sense of how you might apply the Taoist principles and nutrition to your own chart.

Meryl Streep

Meryl Streep is one of the most accomplished actresses of her generation. In Meryl Streep's chart, her water day master is very weak, as are her wood expression and her metal resource. Acting energy is usually connected to fire, and fire is her wealth phase. Your wealth phase is one place where we can find achievements and where you can make money.

Her achievements have come to her from enormous self-discipline. From an early age she taught herself acting and became accomplished in learning her lines and mimicking accents (think of her Danish accent in *Out of Africa* and her British English for *The French Lieutenant's Woman*). Her mother was very encouraging and impressed upon her that she could do anything she put her mind to. This attitude has stayed with her, and her strong earth power has been the driving force in her success, as well as making her feel that she had the power to do it.

Throughout her career, she has been nominated for more major awards than any other male or female actor and has won eight Golden Globes, three Oscars, and one Cannes Film Festival. So her earth storehouse knows how to fill up. Her strong earth comes over as an intimidating style that some people have found off putting in a woman, but she has persevered. Her earth power is also where her incredible self-discipline and perfectionism come from. For one film she took hours of violin lessons to feel her part, and for another one she learned to play the guitar. She practiced singing Abba songs for *Mama Mia,* and she learned how to sing off-key for her title role in *Florence Foster Jenkins.* She works very hard to be able to portray the essential core of a character.

Her earth sense of fairness and justice is shown through her many philanthropic projects connected with scholarships, feminism, equal rights, theaters, spreading female empowerment, and even funding a screenwriters' writing lab for female screenwriters over forty years old. The lower fire and very strong earth means that she leads a fairly unstarlike life, despite her high profile and successes. Earth plays a very

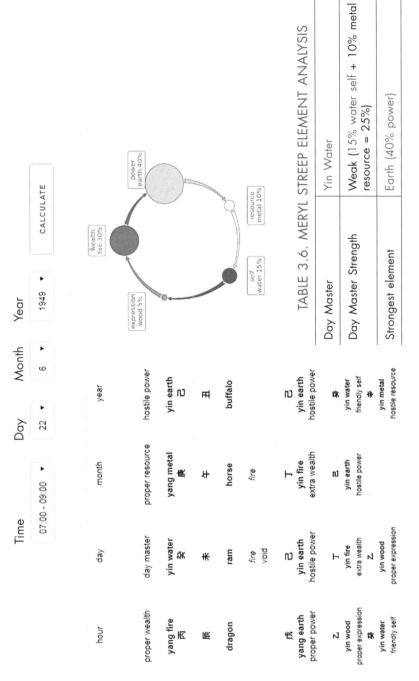

Time	Day	Month	Year
07:00 - 09:00 ▸	22 ▸	6 ▸	1949 ▸

CALCULATE

hour	day	month	year
proper wealth	day master	proper resource	hostile power
yang fire 丙	yin water 癸	yang metal 庚	yin earth 己
辰 dragon	未 ram	午 horse	丑 buffalo
		fire	fire void

power earth 40%

wealth fire 30%

expression wood 5%

self water 15%

resource metal 10%

hour
戊 yang earth proper power
乙 yin wood proper expression
癸 yin water friendly self

day
己 yin earth hostile power
丁 yin fire extra wealth
乙 yin wood proper expression

month
丁 yin fire extra wealth
己 yin earth hostile power

year
己 yin earth hostile power
癸 yin water friendly self
辛 yin metal hostile resource

TABLE 3.6. MERYL STREEP ELEMENT ANALYSIS

Day Master	Yin Water
Day Master Strength	Weak (15% water self + 10% metal resource = 25%)
Strongest element	Earth (40% power)

Fig. 3.4. Meryl Streep's five-element makeup and natal chart

big role in her life, and she could be left with the feeling that her philosophical, touchy-feely water day master is not always allowed out to play. This could be balanced by using Taoist practices as well as an understanding of Taoist nutrition.

Just as with our own charts, we can best apply Meryl Streep's chart by analyzing the strength of her organs. Table 3.7 on page 78 shows the self-calculation organ analysis described on pages 57–60 based on the number of times each yin and yang element appears in her natal chart. Remember that 0 indicates deficient energy, 1 and 2 indicate balanced energy, and 3 (or more) indicates high or excess energy. Table 3.8 on page 78 shows her organ analysis based on more complex calculations, which, in addition to counting the yin and yang elements, includes a traditional Chinese medicine calculation that gives the animal branches an extra element. Note that this table is similar, but some values differ. This calculation is too complex for our purposes here, but you can purchase this more in-depth chart for your own organ analysis on the Universal Healing Tao Inner Alchemy website.

Based on her chart and the balance of her elements, Meryl Streep would benefit from doing the spleen and heart Healing Sounds to bring down those dominating earth and fire energies. With the Inner Smile she could boost her day master water energy, smiling balance into the strong elements to boost both her metal and water. With five-element nutrition she could better support her gallbladder and bladder energy. She should avoid the cool and cold foods from the gallbladder and bladder lists because cooling foods decrease chi. At the same time, she could avoid the hot foods on the spleen list, because she already has excess chi in the spleen. But she has many well-balanced, for yin and yang, organ energies in her lungs, large intestine, stomach, and small intestine.

Looking at her pictogram and the family and phase interactions of her chart, she may want to strengthen her day master by eating water and metal foods. Water is her resource, which feeds her day master. Because earth is so strong in her chart, she may want to avoid overdoing foods on the earth list as well as sweet foods (earth's flavor).

TABLE 3.7. MERYL STREEP'S ORGAN ANALYSIS

Based on Her Basic Natal Chart (Fig. 3.4)

ELEMENT	ORGAN	VALUE
Yin Fire	Heart	2
Yang Fire	Small intestine	1
Yin Earth	Spleen, pancreas	3
Yang Earth	Stomach	1
Yin Metal	Lungs	1
Yang Metal	Large intestine	1
Yin Water	Kidneys	3
Yang Water	Bladder	0
Yin Wood	Liver	2
Yang Wood	Gallbladder	0

TABLE 3.8. MERYL STREEP'S IN-DEPTH ORGAN ANALYSIS

ELEMENT	ORGAN	VALUE
FIRE	Heart, pericardium	2
FIRE	Small intestine, triple warmer	1
EARTH	Spleen, pancreas	4
EARTH	Stomach	2
METAL	Lungs	1
METAL	Large intestine	1
WATER	Kidneys	3
WATER	Bladder	0
WOOD	Liver	3
WOOD	Gallbladder	0

What is most important is that she looks at her chart as a whole to be sure that her work to balance one element or organ doesn't bring imbalance to another aspect of her chart and in turn to her self.

Barack Obama

Former president Barack Obama is a strong yin earth day master; his day master plus his fire resources make up 58 percent of his five-element energy, so he is a strong, self-assured person.

A politician's caring qualities and connection with the people can be tracked by their quality and quantity of earth and in what position in their five phases it is found. Because earth is usually about people, society, fairness, and justice, a chart such as Barack Obama's shows that he wanted to make changes to better the greater population's lives during his presidency. Expressing his earth values gave him the push to succeed in politics and achieve the milestone of being the first nonwhite president of the United States.

Barack Obama's lowest element is his water element. His day master is much stronger than the wood power element, so he can use politics and his power phase for his deeper goals, rather than its using him. Wood played a significant part in his life; it is the energy of a lawyer. Studying and practicing law structured much of his life, including his work to have the Affordable Care Act, or "Obamacare," a plan for health care and health insurance for all, passed by a reluctant legislature. Wood, and especially yin wood, is important to the chart as it is the *yong shen,* the very favorable energy that keeps his strong day master in check, the grandparent energy to his day master, bringing it more in balance within the chart. His stability is due to the wood's keeping him structured. His chart reflects the deep bond he had with his grandmother, with whom he lived in Hawaii while his mother was working as an anthropologist in Indonesia. Wood is also the day master energy of his wife, Michelle Obama, so we can say that both his wife and wood power phase give him great support.

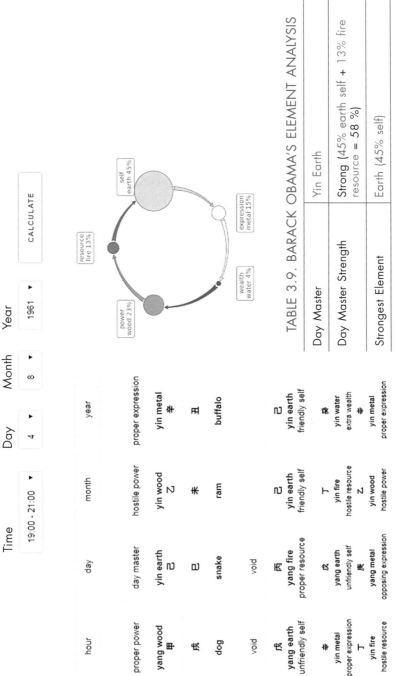

Time   Day   Month   Year

19:00 - 21:00 ▾   4 ▾   8 ▾   1961 ▾   CALCULATE

	hour	day	month	year
	proper power	day master	hostile power	proper expression
	yang wood 甲	yin earth 己	yin wood 乙	yin metal 辛
	戌	巳	未	丑
	dog	snake	ram	buffalo
	void	void		
	戌 yang earth unfriendly self	丙 yang fire proper resource	己 yin earth friendly self	己 yin earth friendly self
	辛 yin metal proper expression	戊 yang earth unfriendly self	丁 yin fire hostile resource	癸 yin water extra wealth
	丁 yin fire hostile resource	庚 yang metal opposing expression	乙 yin wood hostile power	辛 yin metal proper expression

self earth 45%

resource fire 13%

expression metal 15%

power wood 23%

wealth water 4%

TABLE 3.9. BARACK OBAMA'S ELEMENT ANALYSIS

Day Master	Yin Earth
Day Master Strength	Strong (45% earth self + 13% fire resource = 58 %)
Strongest Element	Earth (45% self)

Fig. 3.5. Barack Obama's five-element makeup and natal chart

On page 83 are the organ analysis tables for both Barack and Michelle Obama (see tables 3.11 and 3.12). It is generally easier for a couple to eat the same things. If we look for similarities in the organ analysis charts of Barack and Michelle Obama, they both have balanced heart energy and could both decide to work on reducing spleen and pancreas energy. However, they would want to be careful not to reduce bladder energy for Barack and gallbladder, stomach, and small intestine energy for Michelle. As these organs are all fairly balanced in the partner's chart, a slight increase in these foods for both should not upset the overall balance.

Both would need to add cool or cold foods from the spleen and pancreas list to decrease their excessive chi in these organs. Barack could also benefit from cool and cold lungs foods, and Michelle could create more balance by adding cool and cold foods for the liver and kidneys. Similar to Meryl Streep, Barack would want to limit sweet foods in his diet, as his earth element is already quite strong, and he might add more foods from the water list, as well as salty foods to bolster his weak water. However, Michelle's water is quite strong and is feeding her already strong wood day master, so she would want to hold back on the salty foods.

Another way to create balance is to refer back to figs. 2.6 and 2.7 (pages 42 and 43) and look at the times of day when we receive the missing energies we are trying to enhance from this couple's charts: gallbladder 11:00 p.m. to 1:00 a.m., large intestine 5:00 a.m. to 7:00 a.m., stomach 7:00 a.m. to 9:00 a.m., small intestine 1:00 p.m. to 3:00 p.m., and bladder 3:00 to 5:00 p.m. Gallbladder time should find you in bed, asleep, allowing digestion to work well; it is the wood organs' involvement, meaning early nights in order to be asleep by then. Breakfasting well and in five-color Eastern style during large intestine and stomach times gives digestion another chance to work well. This would also be a good time to practice Taoist exercises to enhance the stomach before breakfast. Good digestion continues during the small intestine time, and the late afternoon would give the couple a great opportunity to get together for some five-element practices or meditations to enhance small intestine and bladder energy as they move into the low digestion phase of the day.

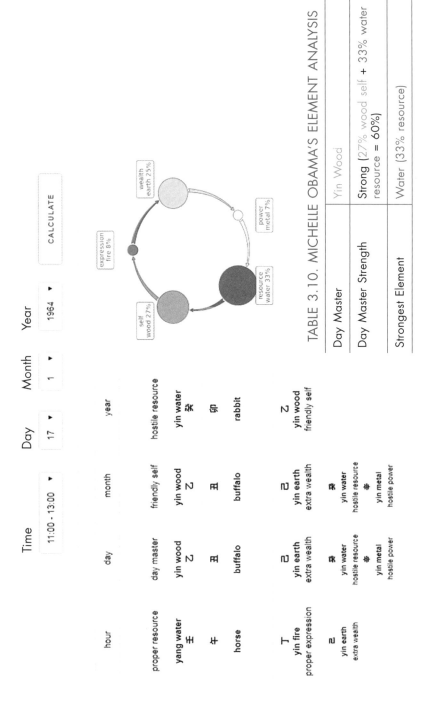

Time: 11:00 - 13:00 ▼   Day: 17 ▼   Month: 1 ▼   Year: 1964 ▼   CALCULATE

	hour	day	month	year
	proper resource	day master	friendly self	hostile resource
	yang water 壬	yin wood 乙	yin wood 乙	yin water 癸
	午	丑	丑	卯
	horse	buffalo	buffalo	rabbit
	丁 yin fire proper expression	己 yin earth extra wealth	己 yin earth extra wealth	乙 yin wood friendly self
	己 yin earth extra wealth	癸 yin water hostile resource	癸 yin water hostile resource	
		辛 yin metal hostile power	辛 yin metal hostile power	

self wood 27%
wealth earth 25%
expression fire 8%
power metal 7%
resource water 33%

TABLE 3.10. MICHELLE OBAMA'S ELEMENT ANALYSIS

Day Master	Yin Wood
Day Master Strength	Strong (27% wood self + 33% water resource = 60%)
Strongest Element	Water (33% resource)

Fig. 3.6 Michelle Obama's five-element makeup and natal chart

TABLE 3.11. BARACK OBAMA'S ORGAN ANALYSIS

Based on His Basic Natal Chart (Fig. 3.5)

ELEMENT	ORGAN	VALUE
Yin Fire	Heart	2
Yang Fire	Small intestines	1
Yin Earth	Spleen, pancreas	3
Yang Earth	Stomach	2
Yin Metal	Lungs	3
Yang Metal	Large intestine	1
Yin Water	Kidneys	1
Yang Water	Bladder	0
Yin Wood	Liver	2
Yang Wood	Gallbladder	1

TABLE 3.12. MICHELLE OBAMA'S ORGAN ANALYSIS

Based on Her Basic Natal Chart (Fig. 3.6)

ELEMENT	ORGAN	VALUE
Yin Fire	Heart	1
Yang Fire	Small intestine	0
Yin Earth	Spleen, pancreas	3
Yang Earth	Stomach	0
Yin Metal	Lungs	2
Yang Metal	Large intestine	0
Yin Water	Kidneys	3
Yang Water	Bladder	1
Yin Wood	Liver	3
Yang Wood	Gallbladder	0

Paul McCartney

Paul McCartney is considered one of the most successful composers/ performers in music; he has been knighted by the queen and has acquired a lot of wealth. He is a weak yang water day master with strong fire wealth dominant in his chart. With such strong fire, his love of performing is a given, as fire is a performing energy, and that will always be the case for him. His earth power is slightly larger than his day master and so formative. For example, he supports many social causes—an earth trait.

His organ analysis in table 3.14 on page 86 shows that many areas need balancing. You can see that his fire—wealth—is high in his pictogram and, although balanced in its yang aspect, has excessive yin heart energy. Decreasing heart chi with cool and cold foods from that list would create more balance here. Increasing the lungs', large intestine, and kidneys' chi by avoiding cool and cold foods on those lists in favor of warm and hot ones would also be beneficial. Bringing down the spleen and pancreas chi by eating cool foods on that list would help even out his power.

Based on his pictogram and the family and phase interactions of his chart, Paul McCartney may want to give extra attention to water and metal foods, as both are quite weak. He would of course want to keep in mind the balance of his organs within these elements as well. It would be important for him to eat foods from the metal list to increase this nonexistent resource in his natal chart, as well as foods with metal flavors and colors—pungent, hot, white, gold, silver, or bronze. Balancing this metal resource is very important, as it is the resource or support for an already weak water day master. He would also want to add foods from the water list, as well as foods that are salty and black or dark blue. He may also want to lessen the amount of fire foods in his diet to create more balance throughout the elements.

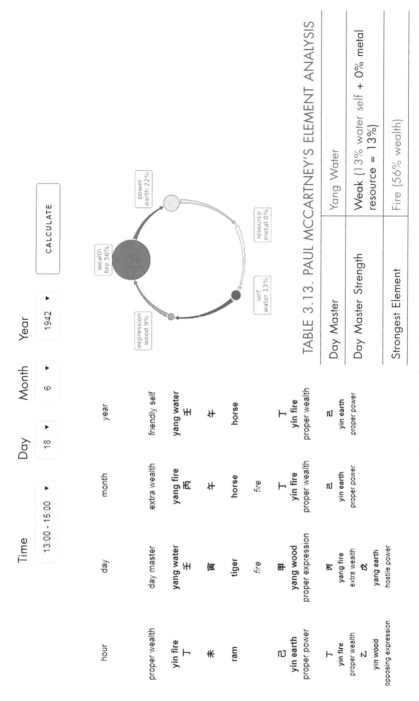

Fig. 3.7. Paul McCartney's five-element makeup and natal chart

TABLE 3.13. PAUL MCCARTNEY'S ELEMENT ANALYSIS

Day Master	Yang Water
Day Master Strength	Weak (13% water self + 0% metal resource = 13%)
Strongest Element	Fire (56% wealth)

TABLE 3.14. PAUL McCARTNEY'S ORGAN ANALYSIS

Based on His Basic Natal Chart (Fig. 3.7)

ELEMENT	ORGAN	VALUE
Yin Fire	Heart	4
Yang Fire	Small intestine	2
Yin Earth	Spleen, pancreas	3
Yang Earth	Stomach	1
Yin Metal	Lungs	0
Yang Metal	Large intestine	0
Yin Water	Kidney	0
Yang Water	Bladder	2
Yin Wood	Liver	1
Yang Wood	Gallbladder	1

You can see in these examples how our theme of the importance of balance becomes tangible—balance of nutritional and physical/mental practices, of flavor and color, of assessing and reassessing our charts based on an understanding of how the organs work together to create a healthy whole.

THE INFLUENCE OF INCOMING ENERGIES

Your astrological pictogram (as calculated on the Universal Healing Tao Inner Alchemy website) is an analysis of what you are born with, beginning with that first gasp of air; it is a calculation of your five-element makeup. Each of the five elements relates to organs, emotions, sense organs, and types of actions in your life on the level of vibrational chi, or vital energy. However, the planets move in the heavens; the universe is not static but constantly changing. From your birth data, Taoist astrology can also calculate when the energies of the five elements will become stronger or weaker in you according to ten-year or annual "luck cycles,"* as these revolving planetary energies are called in Chinese astrology. This kind of more in-depth astrological analysis done by a professional, or visible on the full Inner Alchemy astrology chart, can suggest additional remedies to assist in addressing the changing energies and how they affect your basic elemental makeup.

Luck cycles that occur during early childhood and school years will influence how a person studies and even which subjects she chose to study. For example, an early wood luck cycle can show a good attitude toward learning and success at school. If this luck cycle hits people in middle teenage years, then as well as general interest in studying they might choose law or accountancy, writing, music, art, or another of the typical wood pursuits, thus further shaping their life. Luck cycles will impact your health, wealth, and relationships, so delving further into this information could suggest additional uses of five-element nutrition. By knowing in advance what your luck factors are, you can shape these forces to your advantage, lessening the impact of difficult influences and enhancing the effects of the more favorable energies.

The basic building blocks of the whole cosmos, as well as the human body—the macrocosm and microcosm—are described by the five elements. By studying our natal astrology chart we can see which of our elements need enhancing or weakening. Taoists believe that the elements are expressed in our major organs and that these organs store the negative and positive emotions associated with the five elements. Weak or strong organ energy is a major factor in health, as are the emotions.

---

*For detailed information on how to calculate your luck cycles, as well as other aspects of Chinese astrology, see *Inner Alchemy Astrology: Practical Techniques for Controlling Your Destiny,* by Mantak Chia and Christine Harkness-Giles. To find more in-depth charts or to contact a professional Inner Alchemy astrologer, visit the Universal Healing Tao Inner Alchemy website.

They affect our hormones, immune system, and blood circulation. A diet that is adapted to the five elements will support optimal health and well-being in our organs, in our emotions, and in our beings as a whole. So follow the Taoist advice, include each of the five elements in your diet on a daily basis.

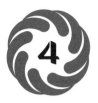

Fire Element

Fire is a radiating and shining energy, and fire is depicted at the top of the five-element pictogram, so we start with this element. The all-important *shen*, a person's spirit, resides in the heart, the principle yin fire organ, while the small intestine is the principle yang fire organ. The blood vessels are considered to be fire, as is the tongue. The following qualities describe a fire day master but would also be felt by you if fire is strong anywhere within the phases of your five-element makeup.

THE QUALITIES OF FIRE

The heart is considered the lord of all the organs, the commander. The heart maintains order and can accept nourishment coming from all parts of the body, as blood flows back into it from the farthest outposts. The heart shines the light of the spirit and radiates this throughout the whole being, so nothing must block this radiance of the spirit. The heart must be calm and peaceful to allow all the transformational processes that make up the life of a human being.

Those with dominant fire must be careful not to let hatred, impatience, and hastiness grow in them. It is very important to eliminate hatred especially, as it is the one emotion that a person passes on to the next generation. Wars and feuds that spread through communities and nations are evidence of how this emotion is passed from one generation to the next. As well as being stored in the heart, it can enter the bones, at which point only a healing touch Taoist massage such as Chi Nei Tsang, as well as meditation, can get rid of it. And of course it is not only those with a fire day master who can feel hatred, as we all have some fire in us. Hastiness and impatience lead to challenging behavior too.

The yin facet of an element is the more subtle, smaller one, and the yang facet is the larger, more noticeable one. Yin fire is glowing moonlight and candles. It is mild, gentle, adventurous, diplomatic, private, conservative, courteous, warm, deep, careful, cautious, and unhurried and pays attention to detail, in contrast to the hotter yang fire. Yin fire day masters are sentimental, inspirational, motivating, giving, good friends, sensitive, tolerant, dependable, good motivators, born leaders, and good performers. They are fast thinkers, taking pride in leading and illuminating others and in careful planning. They can be fickle but know how to rise to any occasion with endurance and energy. Easily demotivated, they do not always communicate their feelings.

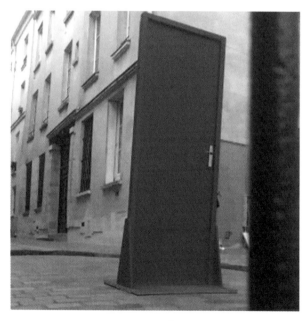

Fig. 4.1. Fire—our door to passion

Yang fire is like the sun—it radiates warmth and light. It can be generous, open, sincere, just, upright, noble, vibrant, explosive, passionate, independent, outgoing, selfish, lonely, arrogant, opinionated, charismatic, larger than life, visible, straightforward, relentless, and bossy. Yang fire day masters are born leaders and warriors, good talkers but not always good listeners. Expressive and sentimental, yang fire day masters will take up a cause with vigor. They like routines but get bored easily or become impatient. These sun kings can think the world revolves around them; although they do think of helping others, they can lose support as a result of their conceitedness and impatience in thought, word, and deed, and this can lead to misunderstandings. They have a tendency to waste resources and suffer from mood swings and bad tempers. They need to keep their flames under control to achieve their potential.

FIRE NUTRITION:
TASTE, SEASON, AND COLOR

Bitter is the taste associated with the element fire. During summer it can be useful to eat more raw food to strengthen the fire organs of the heart and small intestine. Bitter is also the most cooling flavor, excellent for excessive body heat, fever, or just cooling down on a hot summer day.

According to traditional Chinese medicine, bitter flavor is good for regulating body temperature and can help balance out negative effects of an excess of pungent flavor (associated with metal) such as knotted muscles and strain to the liver. However, an excess of bitter flavor can injure the lungs and cause the stomach to become congested. Bitter can be balanced by a moderate amount of salty food (associated with water).

Red, purple, and pink are the colors of fire, and red foods in particular are good for the blood. Purple sweet potatoes, blood oranges, red cabbage, blackberries, blueberries, strawberries, eggplant, red grapes, and plums all owe their color to their content of anthocyanin pigment, and they are fire foods. This pigment releases anti-inflammatory compounds that boost blood flow in the body and brain, helping to forestall many of the aging diseases, such as type 2 diabetes, dementia, and high blood pressure. We see this in "red" drinks made from these foods too, from red wine to black currant syrups. Purple sweet potatoes are one of the staples of the population of Okinawa, considered a "longevity island." Red foods are also sometimes considered the food of love; in any Valentine's Day feast you are likely to find such things as strawberries or pink or red iced cakes, an example of the relationship between the heart fire organ and the color red.

FIRE SUPERFOODS

Adzuki beans help when blood appears in bowel movements and for bleeding during pregnancy.

Artichoke stimulates the flow of bile from the liver while helping to relieve gallstones. It is known as a hangover cure, helps digestion and IBS, and lowers "bad" cholesterol, high blood sugar, and high blood pressure. It also helps water retention and bladder and kidney problems. Artichoke can also be used as a tea for its many health-giving properties.

Asparagus reduces coughing by lubricating the lungs and moving phlegm. It also reduces high blood pressure and helps expel parasites from the digestive tract. It is a natural diuretic and flushes the urinary tract (note that after you eat asparagus, urine will have a distinctive odor).

Blueberries help brain neurons communicate better. They contain compounds that can help prevent mental deterioration, diabetes, cancer, Alzheimer's disease, and heart disease, and they also help eyesight. They are considered useful in antiaging regimes, and they support the digestion and can help in weight loss.

Cacao helps most heart functions and the circulatory system. It is considered a brain and longevity food that improves energy levels, assists in weight loss, and reduces inflammation. It is said to have forty times more antioxidants than blueberries, is the most potent plant-based source of iron, and contains much more calcium than cow's milk. A compound in cacao known as phenylethylamine is a central nervous system stimulant sometimes called the "love drug" because it induces a good mood. It is more potent in its raw form, as heating chocolate destroys some of its valuable nutrients.

Grapefruit has been identified as a superfood for so long now that there was once a popular one-food diet based on this fruit. A one-food diet is unwise, although grapefruit does have many health-improving attributes. It is good for weight loss by promoting appetite control; it lowers cholesterol and improves heart health; it may reduce the risk of kidney stones; and because it is so hydrating it is good for cleansing and constipation. (Note that many common drugs have negative and sometimes dangerous interactions with grapefruit.)

Thyme is good for coughs and sore throats and has antibacterial properties.

Turmeric is good for energy circulation and lowering menstruation flow, and it has become popularly regarded in the West in recent years as a potent anti-inflammatory.

NUTRITION TO BALANCE FIRE IN YOUR CHART

To begin with you can balance fire in and of itself by looking at your own percentage of the element and adjusting your diet accordingly using both the food tables and the fire nutrition information above. In addition to this, you can look at the family and phase cycles to note what will strengthen weak fire or balance out excessive fire as well as looking at how to balance out the fire organs based on your organ analysis table.

Weak Fire

As we have learned, fire can be weak in comparison to the other percentages on your chart, but it can also be weakened by its relationship to the other elements. If fire is weak in your chart you will likely want to add some additional fire foods to your diet. One simple way to do this is through culinary herbs. Many common culinary herbs are included in the fire list. Using them in cooking has the advantages of adding the many health-giving properties they possess and making it easier to have all five elements represented on your plate. Using these culinary herbs can help you adapt a meal so that a nonfire food you may want to eat can better suit your nutritional needs.

If your earth element is quite strong, you may want to add a little extra fire into your diet, as fire feeds earth and may be depleted by an excess of that element. If you have an excess of wood in your chart, you may not need to focus as much on increasing fire foods, even if fire is fairly weak, because wood is the parent that feeds fire.

Excessive Fire

If you have an excess of fire in your chart, you may want to think about strengthening the element that fire feeds—earth. This will be particularly true if both wood (fire's parent) *and* fire are strong in your chart, so more earth would ensure better chi flow around the elements in the direction of the creating cycle. In addition to being careful not to overdo the amount of fire foods in your diet, you can also look at the nutrition suggestions and food tables in the earth chapter.

Yin and Yang Fire Organs

As we have seen in the previous chapters, whether you have yin or yang fire in your chart is reflected in the yin organ, heart, and the yang organ, small intestines. As well as balancing the elements within you, it is also beneficial to balance the yin and yang within you. So look back at your organ analysis table (see pages 57–60 for how to complete this table based on your individual chart) to get an idea of the balance of your fire organs. Remember that 0 indicates deficient energy, 1 and 2 indicate balanced energy, and 3 (or more) indicate high or excess energy.

If either the yin or yang polarity of fire is absent from your chart or heavily outbalanced by the other (by two or more), this could indicate that the organ energy associated with that polarity is weak, or at least dominated by the other polarity's organ. Finding warm or hot foods for the weak organ in the fire food tables can help strengthen it, as can consuming cool or cold foods for the dominant organ.

If the energy is excessive or very weak, remember that this will also play on your emotions (see table 1.1 on page 17). For example, many occurrences of yang or yin fire in your chart will make the negative emotions of fire quite likely—impatience, hastiness, and so on. In TCM, excesses or deficiencies indicate issues, so a very weak element would also suggest sensitivities around these emotions. Remember also that the heart sound, one of the Six Healing Sounds described on pages 22 to 27 will help balance this. If the organ energy is very strong, doing the sounds has the double advantage of calming those negative emotions associated with it but also making room for positive emotions when releasing the negative ones. The Tao is all about balance, and Taoists want to treat the five flavors, colors, and elements as if they were your children every day and give them a bit of presence on your plate.

FIRE ELEMENT AND ORGAN FOOD TABLES

The temperature column means that the food "cools" (cool/cold), or *diminishes,* the chi for the noted organ(s) or "warms/heats" (warm/hot), or *increases,* the chi. So remember that if you want to increase energy for the given organ, then avoid cool or cold foods and favor warm or hot ones. If you have excessive energy, then you want to avoid warm and hot foods and favor cool or cold ones. If you are treating several organs at the same time, you will want to watch for foods that are good for one yet not good for another organ. In that case, we prefer to first work on an organ that has no energy appearing for it in the natal chart, then treat the very high energy ones, and so on, in descending order. Neutral foods have neither effect and can be eaten in any scenario.

Remember also that fire organ's chi can be boosted by pungent foods (metal's flavor) as fire controls metal; it is a wealth for them, but too much can be overwhelming. Fire organs can also benefit from sour foods (wood's flavor), as fire is nourished and fed by wood. Fire is weakened by earth, so too many sweet foods are not good for weak fire organs, but good to calm down excessive fire energy. Water controls fire and so eating too many salty or water foods can put adverse control on the fire organs. But it all depends on quantity! Whatever your required balance for harmony in your own elements, remember to eat all the five elements and colors every day!

TABLE 4.1. FOODS THAT SUPPORT FIRE ORGANS AND HEALTH

FOOD	FLAVOR(S)	TEMPERATURE	YIN ORGAN	YANG ORGAN
Adzuki bean	Sweet, sour	Neutral	Heart	Small intestine
Aloe vera	Bitter	Neutral	Heart	
Artichoke	Sweet, salty, bitter	Cool	Heart	
Asparagus	Sweet, bitter	Cold		Small intestine
Banana	Sweet	Cold	Heart	Small intestine
Basil	Sweet, pungent, bitter	Warm	Heart	
Blueberry	Sour	Cool	Heart	
Cabbage	Sweet	Cool		Small intestine
Cauliflower	Sour	Cool	Heart	Small intestine
Cacao	Bitter, sweet	Warm	Heart	Small intestine
Chickpea	Sweet	Neutral	Heart	Small intestine
Eggplant	Sweet	Cool	Heart	
Onion	Pungent, sweet	Warm	Heart	Small intestine
Pepper (chili)	Pungent	Hot	Heart	
Plum (Victoria, European, sweet, and purple)	Sweet, sour	Warm	Heart	Small intestine

TABLE 4.1. FOODS THAT SUPPORT
FIRE ORGANS AND HEALTH (cont.)

FOOD	FLAVOR(S)	TEMPERATURE	YIN ORGAN	YANG ORGAN
Pomegranate	Sweet, sour	Neutral	Heart	
Rosemary	Sweet, pungent	Warm	Heart	
Saffron	Pungent	Neutral	Heart	
Sage	Pungent	Warm		
Scallion	Sweet, bitter	Warm	Heart	
Seaweed	Sweet, salty	Cool	Heart	Small intestine
Spinach	Sweet	Cool		Small intestine
Tomato (red)	Sweet, sour	Warm (when sweet and ripe)		Small intestine
Thyme	Pungent, bitter	Warm	Heart	
Turmeric	Pungent, bitter	Warm	Heart	

TABLE 4.2. HEART FOODS

FOOD	FLAVOR(S)	TEMPERATURE
Adzuki bean	Sweet, sour	Neutral
Almond	Sweet	Neutral
Aloe vera	Bitter	Neutral
Aniseed	Sweet, pungent	Warm
Apple	Sweet, sour	Cool
Cherry	Sweet	Warm
Chickpea	Sweet	Neutral
Chili	Pungent	Hot
Cinnamon (twig)	Sweet, pungent	Warm
Garlic	Sweet, pungent, salty	Hot
Hawthorn	Sweet, sour	Warm
Lentil	Sweet	Neutral
Licorice	Sweet	Neutral

TABLE 4.2. HEART FOODS (cont.)

FOOD	FLAVOR(S)	TEMPERATURE
Marjoram	Sweet, pungent	Cool
Mung bean	Sweet	Cool
Pepper (black)	Sweet, pungent	Hot
Persimmon	Sweet	Cold
Pollen	Sweet, pungent, salty, sour, bitter	Neutral
Rosemary	Sweet, pungent	Warm
Saffron	Pungent	Neutral
Scallion	Pungent, bitter	Warm
Watermelon	Sweet	Cold
Wheat germ	Pungent	Cold

TABLE 4.3. SMALL INTESTINE FOODS

FOODS	FLAVOR(S)	TEMPERATURE
Adzuki bean	Sweet, sour	Neutral
Licorice	Sweet	Neutral
Mushroom (button)	Sweet	Cool
Peach	Sweet, sour	Warm
Pepper (white)	Pungent, bitter	Hot
Plantain	Sweet	Cold
Pollen	Sweet, pungent, salty, sour, bitter	Neutral
Salt	Salty	Cold
Spinach	Sweet	Cool
Tamarind	Sweet, sour	Cool
Wheat germ	Pungent	Cold

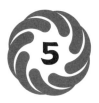

Earth Element

The spleen and pancreas are yin earth organs, and the stomach is a yang earth organ, while the flesh and the mouth are the earth sensory organs. The principle earth organs are literally warehouses of energy—they store and distribute, receive and redistribute food. The qualities of the earth organs are reflected in the qualities of those who are predominantly earth people.

QUALITIES OF EARTH

Earth people have a strong sense of fairness and justice, but trust is always an issue for earth people, and negative energies can bring on major attacks of worry and anxiety. If they do not have so much fire in their chart such that the heat of fire's charisma overwhelms their basic earthiness, they will get their mission accomplished in a steady and consistent style. They can take their time and organize with flair and brilliance; they are happy with change as long as they can go into it with their planned-for-perfection earthy approach. They are the managers and the human resource experts.

Those with yin earth traits will have a versatile intellect, a good and rapid grasp of knowledge, and an easy understanding of concepts (making for good students and teachers). They are innovative, productive, hardworking, resourceful, creative, sensitive, intuitive, good-hearted, dependable, and driven to self-improvement. They have a strong sense of justice and fairness, empathy for others, and an understanding of others' failings and weaknesses. They are not floored by problems and difficulties and are sensitive to energy waves. However, they can also lack adaptability and spontaneity, worry too much, and let anxiety sabotage their projects, decisions, and concentration. Their ability to step in and organize and nurture people can mean they are sometimes taken for granted by others.

Those with yang earth traits are protective, loyal, trustworthy, caring, dependable, solid, stubborn, steady, broad-minded, fair, honest, unwavering, stable, self-respecting, willful, and slow to gain momentum. They can be inspiring to others, do not easily lose sight of their goal, and know how to get down to the nitty-gritty in any task. They have high notions of justice and fairness, as well as organizational skills. Their tendency to be inflexible and their chronic worrying can sometimes compromise their projects. Yang earth is the energy of round-topped mountains rather than angular-topped ones (which are shaped by fire), whereas yin earth is the fertile, moist soil of the garden, which can be easily washed away in the rain and needs plants or trees to protect it. Yin earth can be much more flexible and responsive to change than yang earth.

Earth is the spirit of intention; directionally, its energy comes from the center of the elements. This is a grounded and focused energy that can get down to brass tacks. The versatility of the earth element along with the managing skills associated with the earth element means that earth people can mimic the other elemental traits to accomplish a task, whereas the other four energies are more specifically targeted. For this reason we find earth people have a greater variety of roles and more of an ability to change career paths than the other four elements. It is rare to find earth people in careers and positions that are not connected with people. They make excellent managers of people, companies, and systems. They are good in construction and land matters; earth is the basis of so many building materials in our civilization. The shape of this form of energy is considered to be rectangular or square. Because of their sense of fairness and justice, they have the energy to be good judges, attorneys, and social workers. Their organizational skills and social interests mean that we often have earth day master politicians, although usually on the Democratic, Socialist, or Left side of the political spectrum. Earth, when combined with strong wood, makes for super organizational skills, as wood adds its planning and visionary energy to earth qualities.

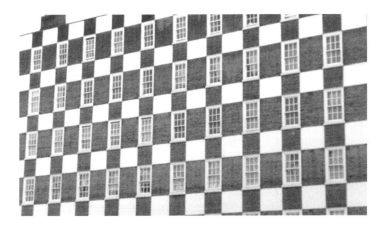

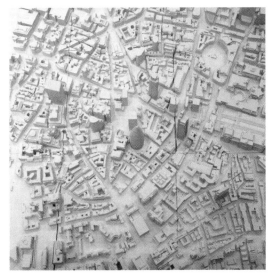

Fig. 5.1. Earth provides the building blocks of our civilization.

EARTH NUTRITION:
TASTE, SEASON, AND COLOR

Because earth is at the center of the four elements, it is our principal connection to planet Earth. This is why there are many more earth foods than those belonging to the other elements. The taste of earth is sweet, which has an uplifting and drying effect. The sweetness of maternal milk is our first taste sensation as a baby, and more foods are classified as sweet or earthy in terms of taste than any of the other four flavors. Our taste for sweetness has been abused by the corporate food industry's efforts to maximize their profits by appealing to people's sweet tooth. White refined sugar in particular has caused many health problems, including obesity and diabetes. Sugar should be regarded as a drug with the same addictive qualities as other drugs. As well, processed foods often have sugar disguised by such names as *fructose, corn fructose, corn fructose syrup, maize syrup,* and *glucose syrup.* Considering how harmful these artificial sweeteners are, it's highly questionable that they've been added to meats and vegetable dishes, sauces, condiments, and peanuts and in huge quantities to breakfast cereals. These highly addictive sweeteners lead to overeating and many forms of sickness. Artificial sweeteners are particularly nasty—they are acid-forming and feed cancer.

Enjoying the flavor of naturally sweet earth foods, a principle of food alchemy, is far better than adding these dangerous refined sugars and artificial sweeteners. Paying attention to the quantity and quality of earth element foods is important when addressing weight problems, as so much of the digestive system is of the earth element. And we should not avoid earth foods altogether even if we're trying to lose weight, as we need all the five flavors, and we need to keep our earth organs healthy for them to work properly. Both an excess and a lack of sweet food can injure the earth organs of the stomach, spleen, and pancreas. These organs, of course, impact other parts and systems of the body, such as the pancreas and insulin production, so their importance in food processing is enormous, as is choosing the foods to best look after them. Avoiding bad sugars and artificial sweeteners added in excessive amounts to virtually all prepared foods is more than desirable.

Earth is the energy of the "Indian" summer and the other in-between seasons. Like the seasons it represents, earth is an energy that bridges seasons; it can therefore be applied to most things and as such is spread out throughout the year. The sweet flavor of earth has a retarding effect required at all times, so it too is useful throughout the year. Eating more stewed food during the late summer earth season can help strengthen the stomach, spleen, and pancreas.

Yellow, orange, beige, and brown are the colors of earth. Foods with yellow and orange pigments, such as carrots, sweet potatoes, and apricots, often contain beta-carotene, a strong antioxidant preventive in cancer, blood pressure problems, rheumatoid arthritis, and more.

EARTH SUPERFOODS

Avocados contain oleic acid and beta-sitosterol, both of which lower bad cholesterol. They also offer protection for the prostate and contain the antioxidant glutathione, which helps slow down aging, and folate, which reduces the risk of stroke. Lutein protects eyes from age-related problems, and the vitamins and minerals present in this fruit keep the skin lubricated, bringing a more youthful appearance. Avocado contains 60 percent more potassium than a banana and has natural oils that help restore a natural glow to the skin and strengthen hair.

Bananas are high in potassium and fiber. They lubricate the lungs, lower high blood pressure, and relieve muscle aches by maintaining balance at a cellular level. They merit superfood status, as they are readily available and easy to eat; therefore, a worthwhile snack when on the run and feeling weak.

Buckwheat is an ancient grain that moves energy down the body; therefore, it relieves swelling and reduces heat in the digestive system, stemming diarrhea. Buckwheat is good for skin conditions and high blood pressure, reduces "bad" cholesterol, prevents gallstones, and can be used externally in poultices to stop bleeding and heal wounds. Fiber rich, it also helps in weight control.

Quinoa fits in well with a gluten-free diet and is therefore a good cereal for people with celiac disease or who have a low tolerance to gluten. It has more protein than wheat or rice, and like sweet potatoes it has a low glycemic index, making it particularly good for those with diabetes or hypoglycemia, or for those trying to lose weight. Quinoa is also a good source of calcium, folate, zinc, and other essential minerals that are needed for good skin, hair, and a healthy heart.

Sesame improves blood and strengthens the internal organs. It has a reputation for improving longevity as well as eye, ear, and brain functions. It also helps prevent cardiac problems and lowers bad cholesterol.

Sweet potatoes are low in fat, have a low glycemic index, and are high in fiber. They have anti-inflammatory properties, helping conditions such as colon cancer, asthma, osteoarthritis, lung diseases, colon and stomach ulcers, atherosclerosis, and rheumatoid arthritis.

Watermelon reduces fever and disperses heat, relieving the digestive system. It is also good for the respiratory and cardiovascular systems, and for blood pressure. Watermelon is thirst quenching and cooling in hot weather.

NUTRITION TO BALANCE EARTH IN YOUR CHART

First look at the percentage of earth in your chart, and use the nutrition information above and the food tables below to make adjustments to your diet. Then examine your earth percentage in relation to the other elements in your chart to note what will strengthen weakness or balance out excess.

Weak Earth

If earth is weak in your chart you will likely want to add some additional earth foods to your diet. Like the multidisciplined earth element, earth foods fall into many categories—vegetables, grains, meats, fruits, spices, and herbs—and as noted above make up the longest and most varied list. So it shouldn't be too difficult to add some to your diet.

If your metal element is quite strong, you may want to add a little extra earth into your diet, whether earth is already strong or not. Earth feeds metal and may be depleted by an excess of that element. But adding too much earth will also boost metal whether it is strong or weak. If you have an excess of fire in your chart, you may not need to focus as much on increasing earth foods, even if earth is fairly weak, because fire is feeding it.

Excessive Earth

If you have an excess of earth in your chart, you will want to be especially careful about eating refined sugars. In addition to its effects on the earth organs, an excess of sweet may also injure the kidneys or cause aching bones. It can be balanced by a moderate amount of sour food (associated with wood), but always harmonize by adding fire too. You can also tame excess earth by strengthening metal, the element earth feeds, which in turn weakens earth. In addition to being careful not to overdo the amount of earth foods and sweet flavors in your diet, you can also balance excess earth energy by incorporating foods and nutrition suggestions from the wood and metal chapters.

Yin and Yang Earth Organs

Look at the explanation on pages 94 and 95 in the fire chapter, and use the same formula to determine whether the yin (spleen and pancreas) and yang (stomach) earth organs are deficient or excessive.

The pancreas has an endocrine function, as it releases some

hormones into the blood system and also digestive enzymes; all three of the earth organs are very important, so excessive or deficient earth needs to be monitored. One important example is that if you are looking at diabetes or prediabetic conditions, it is always worth considering how your astrological disposition of earth could be affecting such problems.

EARTH ELEMENT AND ORGAN FOOD TABLES

See the Fire Element and Organ Food Tables section on page 95 to review how to use the temperature column for elemental and organ balance.

Remember also that earth organs can benefit from salty foods (water's flavor), as earth controls water, but too much can be overwhelming. Earth organs can also benefit from bitter foods (fire's flavor), as earth is nourished by fire. Earth is weakened by metal, so too many pungent foods are not good for weak earth organs, but good to calm down excessive earth energy. Wood controls earth, so eating too many sour foods can put adverse control on the earth organs. But it all depends on quantity! Whatever your required balance for harmony in your own elements, remember to eat all the five elements and colors every day!

TABLE 5.1. FOODS THAT SUPPORT EARTH ORGANS AND HEALTH

FOOD	FLAVOR(S)	TEMPERATURE	YIN ORGANS	YANG ORGAN
Alfalfa seed	Bitter	Cool	Spleen, pancreas	Stomach
Alfalfa sprout	Salty, bitter	Cool	Spleen, pancreas	Stomach
Aloe vera	Bitter	Neutral	Spleen, pancreas	Stomach
Apricot	Sweet, sour	Neutral	Spleen, pancreas	
Avocado	Sweet	Cool	Spleen, pancreas	
Banana	Sweet	Cold	Spleen, pancreas	Stomach

TABLE 5.1. FOODS THAT SUPPORT
EARTH ORGANS AND HEALTH (cont.)

FOOD	FLAVOR(S)	TEMPERATURE	YIN ORGANS	YANG ORGAN
Beef	Sweet	Neutral	Spleen, pancreas	Stomach
Black pepper	Sweet, pungent	Hot		Stomach
Blueberry	Sour	Cool	Spleen, pancreas	Stomach
Buckwheat	Sweet	Cool	Spleen, pancreas	Stomach
Carrot	Sweet	Neutral	Spleen, pancreas	
Cauliflower	Sour	Cool	Spleen, pancreas	Stomach
Celery	Sweet, bitter	Cool	Spleen, pancreas	Stomach
Cherry	Sweet	Warm	Spleen, pancreas	Stomach
Chicken	Sweet	Warm	Spleen, pancreas	Stomach
Coriander (leaf)	Pungent	Warm	Spleen, pancreas	
Cucumber	Sweet	Cool	Spleen, pancreas	Stomach
Eggs (chicken)	Sweet	Warm		Stomach
Fig (fresh or dried)	Sweet	Cool	Spleen, pancreas	Stomach
Garlic	Sweet, pungent, salty	Hot	Spleen, pancreas	Stomach
Grape	Sweet, sour	Warm	Spleen, pancreas	
Green bean (string bean)	Sweet	Neutral	Spleen, pancreas	Stomach
Jasmine	Sweet, pungent	Warm	Spleen, pancreas	
Kale	Sweet, bitter	Warm		Stomach
Millet	Sweet, salty	Cool	Spleen, pancreas	Stomach
Oat	Sweet	Warm	Spleen, pancreas	Stomach
Parsley	Pungent, salty, bitter	Warm		Stomach

TABLE 5.1. FOODS THAT SUPPORT
EARTH ORGANS AND HEALTH (cont.)

FOOD	FLAVOR(S)	TEMPERATURE	YIN ORGANS	YANG ORGAN
Parsnip	Sweet, pungent	Warm	Spleen, pancreas	
Quinoa (white)	Sweet, sour	Warm		Stomach
Radish	Pungent, sweet	Cool		Stomach
Rosemary	Sweet, pungent	Warm	Spleen, pancreas	
Sesame oil	Sweet, pungent	Cool		Stomach
Sweet potato	Sweet	Neutral	Spleen, pancreas	
Tomato	Sweet, sour	Cold		Stomach
Watermelon	Sweet	Cold		Stomach

TABLE 5.2. SPLEEN AND PANCREAS FOODS

FOOD	FLAVOR(S)	TEMPERATURE
Almonds	Sweet	Neutral
Aloe vera	Bitter	Neutral
Aniseed	Sweet, pungent	Warm
Avocado	Sweet	Cool
Barley	Sweet, salty	Cool
Beef	Sweet	Neutral
Buckwheat	Sweet	Cool
Caraway	Sweet, pungent	Warm
Carp	Sweet	Neutral
Carrot	Sweet	Neutral
Cayenne	Pungent	Hot

TABLE 5.2. SPLEEN AND PANCREAS FOODS (cont.)

FOOD	FLAVOR(S)	TEMPERATURE
Celery	Sweet, bitter	Cool
Chamomile	Sweet, bitter	Cool
Cherry	Sweet	Warm
Chicken	Sweet	Warm
Chili	Pungent	Hot
Chinese date (red, black, jujube)	Sweet	Neutral
Cinnamon (bark)	Pungent, bitter	Hot
Clove	Pungent	Warm
Coriander (leaf)	Pungent	Warm
Cucumber	Sweet	Cool
Cumin	Pungent	Warm
Dandelion (leaf and root)	Sweet, salty, bitter	Cold
Dill seed	Pungent	Warm
Dongui	Sweet, pungent	Warm
Eggplant	Sweet	Cool
Fennel seed	Sweet, pungent	Warm
Flax	Sweet	Neutral
Garlic	Sweet, pungent, salty	Hot
Ginger (dry)	Pungent	Hot
Ginger (fresh)	Pungent	Warm
Ginseng (American)	Sweet, bitter	Neutral
Ginseng (Chinese)	Sweet	Warm
Glutinous rice (sweet rice)	Sweet	Warm
Grapes	Sweet, sour	Warm
Hawthorn	Sweet, sour	Warm

TABLE 5.2. SPLEEN AND PANCREAS FOODS (cont.)

FOOD	FLAVOR(S)	TEMPERATURE
Hawthorn (berry)	Sweet, sour	Cool
Herring	Sweet	Neutral
Honey	Sweet	Neutral
Juniper	Sweet, pungent, bitter	Warm
Kumquat	Pungent, sweet	Warm
Kuzu	Sweet	Cool
Lamb	Sweet	Hot
Leek	Pungent	Warm
Lentil	Sweet	Neutral
Licorice	Sweet	Neutral
Linseed	Sweet	Neutral
Mandarin orange	Sweet, sour	Cold
Marjoram	Sweet, pungent	Cool
Millet	Sweet, salty	Cool
Mushroom (button)	Sweet	Cool
Nettle	Sweet, salty	Cool
Nutmeg	Pungent	Warm
Oat	Sweet	Warm
Papaya	Sweet, bitter	Neutral
Pea	Sweet	Cool
Peanut oil	Sweet	Neutral
Peppermint	Sweet, pungent	Cool
Persimmon	Sweet	Cold
Pollen	Sweet, pungent, salty, sour, bitter	Neutral
Pork	Sweet, salty	Neutral

TABLE 5.2. SPLEEN AND PANCREAS FOODS (cont.)

FOOD	FLAVOR(S)	TEMPERATURE
Potato	Sweet	Neutral
Pumpkin	Sweet	Neutral
Pumpkin seed	Sweet, bitter	Neutral
Quince	Sour	Warm
Rice	Sweet	Neutral
Rosemary	Sweet, pungent	Warm
Rye	Bitter	Neutral
Salmon	Sweet	Neutral
Sardine	Sweet, salty	Neutral
Sorghum	Sweet	Warm
Spelt	Sweet	Warm
Squash	Sweet	Warm
Star anise	Sweet, pungent	Warm
Strawberry	Sweet, sour	Cool
Sunflower seed	Sweet	Neutral
Swiss chard	Sweet	Cool
Taro root	Sweet, pungent	Neutral
Thyme	Pungent, bitter	Warm
Watercress	Pungent, bitter	Warm

TABLE 5.3. STOMACH FOODS

FOOD	FLAVOR(S)	TEMPERATURE
Apple	Sweet, sour	Cool
Bamboo shoot	Sweet	Cold
Barley	Sweet, salty	Cool
Beef	Sweet	Neutral

TABLE 5.3. STOMACH FOODS (cont.)

FOOD	FLAVOR(S)	TEMPERATURE
Buckwheat	Sweet	Cool
Cayenne	Pungent	Hot
Celery	Sweet, bitter	Cool
Cherry	Sweet	Warm
Chestnut	Sweet	Warm
Chicken	Sweet	Warm
Chickpea	Sweet	Neutral
Chive	Pungent	Warm
Clam (saltwater)	Salty	Cold
Clove	Pungent	Warm
Coriander (seed)	Pungent, sour	Neutral
Cucumber	Sweet	Cool
Eggplant	Sweet	Cool
Fungus (black)	Sweet	Neutral
Garlic	Sweet, pungent, salty	Hot
Ginger (dry)	Pungent	Hot
Ginseng (American)	Sweet, bitter	Neutral
Glutinous rice (sweet rice)	Sweet	Warm
Grapefruit	Sweet, sour	Cold
Horseradish	Pungent	Hot
Kale	Sweet, bitter	Warm
Kuzu	Sweet	Cool
Leek	Pungent	Warm
Lentil	Sweet	Neutral
Lettuce	Sweet, bitter	Cool

TABLE 5.3. STOMACH FOODS (cont.)

FOOD	FLAVOR(S)	TEMPERATURE
Licorice	Sweet	Neutral
Mackerel	Sweet	Neutral
Mango	Sweet, sour	Warm
Millet	Sweet, salty	Cool
Mung bean	Sweet	Cool
Mushroom (button)	Sweet	Cool
Mushroom (Chinese black, shiitake)	Sweet	Neutral
Olive	Sweet, sour	Neutral
Oregano	Sweet, pungent	Warm
Papaya	Sweet, bitter	Neutral
Parsley	Pungent, salty, bitter	Warm
Pea (whole, snow)	Sweet	Cool
Peach	Sweet, sour	Warm
Pear	Sweet, sour	Cool
Pepper (black)	Sweet, pungent	Hot
Pepper (white)	Pungent, bitter	Hot
Pollen	Sweet, pungent, salty, sour, bitter	Neutral
Pork	Sweet, salty	Neutral
Potato	Sweet	Neutral
Radish	Sweet, pungent	Cool
Raspberry (leaf)	Sour	Cool
Rice	Sweet	Neutral
Sage	Pungent	Warm
Salmon	Sweet	Neutral
Salt	Salty	Cold

TABLE 5.3. STOMACH FOODS (cont.)

FOOD	FLAVOR(S)	TEMPERATURE
Sardine	Sweet, salty	Neutral
Seaweed	Salty	Cold
Sesame oil	Sweet, pungent	Cool
Sorghum	Sweet	Warm
Spinach	Sweet	Cool
Squash	Sweet	Warm
Swiss chard	Sweet	Cool
Taro root	Sweet, pungent	Neutral
Tomato	Sweet, sour	Cold
Trout	Sour	Hot
Turmeric	Pungent, bitter	Warm
Turnip	Sweet, pungent, bitter	Neutral
Vinegar	Sour, bitter	Warm
Water chestnut	Sweet	Cold
Watercress	Pungent, bitter	Warm
Watermelon	Sweet	Cold

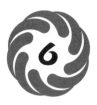

Metal Element

Earth leads us to metal; as earth energy concentrates and crystallizes underground, metal energy is formed. This quality of concentration makes metal energy an analytical power, one of decision making and of processing information to summarize and synthesize it. The yang metal organ is the large intestine and the yin metal organ is the lungs. The metal sense organs are the skin and the nose. Overall, the metal "parts" are the greatest eliminators in the body, and that is why we start the Six Healing Sounds with the lung sound as a detoxification exercise, both on the physical and the emotional plane—from material to immaterial and vice versa, as the Tao says.

THE QUALITIES OF METAL

Although metal is sharp and metal objects are often shaped linearly, such as knives or swords, the shape of metal energy is actually considered to be round; it is the condensing energy of autumn and leads to good analytical and decision-making skills. Metal's energy symbolizes connections in the world as well as networks within the human body, such as the respiratory system. Chi is breathed in directly to the lungs, metal's major yin organ; therefore, sinus, mucus, and other respiratory problems show up when all is not well with one's metal energy. The negative emotions of depression and sadness can reflect the season's progression to the end of the year, or to one's lifetime path. These negative emotions epitomize the problems of not having a proper connection to the universal force; the problems of grief and not letting go show up in the large intestine, the yang metal organ. This important rubbish collector and disposal agent can malfunction, resulting in either diarrhea, which stops proper absorption of nutrients and proper gathering of waste to be eliminated, or constipation, which does the same thing but keeps more toxins in the system. Both conditions indicate a metal imbalance, which is usually seen in the natal astrology (or can be the result of incoming energy cycles as determined by a more detailed astrological reading).

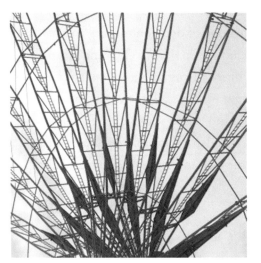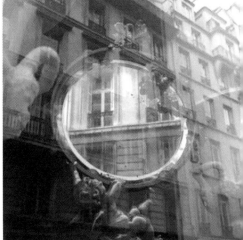

Fig. 6.1. Rounded quality of metal in the wheel and the mirror

As with all five elements, there are both yang and yin aspects. Yang metal is strong and powerful, suitable for swords and weapons with a cutting edge. This quality can show up in metal people as sarcasm, quick wit, fast thinking, and humorous and ironic remarks. Their remarks can be cuttingly blunt, and they therefore can make enemies easily. Beware of verbal barbs, and remember that your words no longer belong to you once they've left your mouth. Yang metal is tough, driven, selfless, righteous, stubborn, direct, sharp, tenacious, determined, loyal, strong willed, and quick witted and does not like to admit to failure. Yang metal day masters have endurance and stamina and can tolerate hands-on work, hardship, and suffering in order to achieve their goals. They know how to build a team, delegate, communicate, analyze a situation, and make executive decisions. They can lack flexibility of thought and attention to detail and can be hasty in action. They show enthusiasm and determination in whatever they do; they may not always express their inner feelings and can therefore appear withdrawn. They are fed by earth and dislike hypocrisy, unfairness, and untruths.

Yin metal is the fine metals used in jewelry, in contrast to the hard sword of yang metal. It is beautiful, gentle, sensitive, attention seeking, sentimental, easily approachable, helpful, expressive, egocentric, opinionated, confident, sharp, driven, quick thinking, moral, attractive and interested in appearances and sociable encounters. Yin metal day masters value relationships and take things such as money at face value. They have fine feelings, unique opinions, and big hearts and can be generous. They want the best. They make good friends but are often on show, seeking the limelight. They love the new, the beautiful, and the latest, and they can seem vain. Their condensing energy means they like to collect, store, and put in the bank—indeed, they are good bankers and good decision makers, are good with money, and have relentless energy for work and projects. This condensing energy means that they do not have space to waste, unlike the storing energy of earth.

Metal people of both polarities can often be found in professions that require rapid analysis and decision making.

METAL NUTRITION: TASTE, SEASON, AND COLOR

The taste associated with metal is variously described as pungent, hot, or spicy. This taste helps clear the respiratory system and expels pathogens

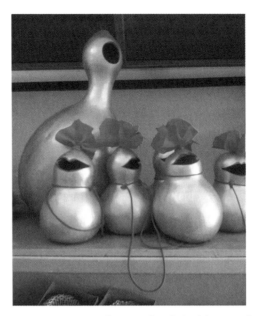

Fig. 6.2. Wu Lou from a dried double gourd
is considered a metal remedy in feng shui and
good for health. Medicine men in ancient China
are often depicted carrying them.

and mucus from the body, making it a good flavor to consume when getting a cold or flu. Ginger, radishes, and many of the spices are metal foods that accomplish this task. Pungent food can help bring balance to spleen and stomach issues, which can be caused by an excess of sour flavor. Both an excess and a lack of pungent food can injure the metal organs of the lungs and large intestine.

Pungent flavor has a dispersing effect particularly needed in metal's autumnal season, just as we disperse the fruits of the fire season as wood is burnt up and the residue minerals taken into the earth. Autumn is a tranquil time of gathering in the harvest. The colors of metal are white, gold, silver, and bronze. In feng shui cures, round objects, circular patterns, and the colors white, gold, silver, and bronze are used where metal is needed, as well as real gold and silver. When it comes to foods, metal colors are integrated through foods such as onion, horseradish, and milk.

METAL SUPERFOODS

Cinnamon regulates the blood, increasing glucose metabolism. It is antioxidant and antimicrobial, reduces "bad" cholesterol and triglycerides, and regulates blood pressure.

Garlic lowers "bad" cholesterol, triglycerides, and blood pressure; has anticoagulants; is antiviral, antiparasitic, and antimicrobial; and has plaque-dissolving properties. Garlic also has a role in preventing common colds and cancer.

Ginger has antioxidants, gingerols, and gingerdiones, making it anti-inflammatory, anticancer, and cholesterol lowering. It is also antiviral, antimicrobial, immune boosting, and blood thinning, and it improves the circulation. Its antinausea properties are particularly good for pregnant women, as it is effective but safe and risk-free during pregnancy. It is good for indigestion and counteracts dampness, promotes chi circulation, and drains water.

Mint is included in many products, including toothpaste, sauces, and chewing gum, confirming that it has superfood status. Ancient wisdom has always known its qualities of decongesting the respiratory system and relieving headaches, indigestion, hay fever, fatigue, and depression. It also helps in preventing cancer and allergies and tonifies the memory and helps in oral hygiene. Mint can prevent homeopathic remedies from working, so it should be avoided in toothpaste and other products when taking them.

Onions are known for easing conditions such as high blood pressure, indigestion, and urine and phlegm problems. It reduces "bad" cholesterol and helps heal wounds as well as urinary and vaginal infections.

Radish counteracts damp, promotes chi circulation, and drains water. It reduces internal heat and inflammation and helps remove toxins from the body. Radish is good for moving mucus in the case of coughs and sinus infections. It is also antitumor. Note that horseradish is the "star" of the radish family.

NUTRITION TO BALANCE METAL IN YOUR CHART

Use the general metal information above and the food tables below to start to balance out the percentage of metal in your makeup. Then integrate your knowledge of the elemental family relationships and phase cycles to note what will nutritionally strengthen weak metal or balance out excessive metal.

Weak Metal

Assess the balance of elements in your chart that can weaken metal—water, which is fed by metal, and wood, metal's grandchild. If these elements, water and wood, are quite strong in your chart, you may want to add a little more metal into your diet, as an excess of these dependent elements deplete metal.

Whether metal is weak on its own or weakened by other elements in your chart, one simple way to add metal to your diet is through spices. Pungent spices such as ginger, cinnamon, cayenne, and oregano can easily be integrated into most dishes. Just as with the culinary herbs of the fire element, using these spices in cooking has the advantage of adding many health-giving properties as well as allowing you to adapt a nonmetal food or meal to increase metal energy.

If you have an excess of earth in your chart, you may not need to focus as much on increasing metal foods, even if metal is fairly weak, because earth feeds metal.

Excessive Metal

If you have an excess of metal in your chart, you may want to think about reversing the strategy above by strengthening the child, water, and the grandchild, wood. This will be particularly true if both metal and metal's parent, earth, are strong in your chart. You can balance out this excess by integrating the nutrition and food suggestions in the water and wood chapters. Also, an excess of pungent flavor can cause liver damage, slow the pulse, and cause weak fingernails and toenails. It can be balanced by a moderate amount of bitter food (associated with fire).

Yin and Yang Metal Organs

Look at the explanation on page 94 in the fire chapter, and use the same formula to determine whether the yin (lungs) and yang (large intestine) metal organs are deficient or excessive.

The metal organs are the main eliminators in our body systems. As well as breathing in oxygen and sending it to be distributed in the body, gas exchange takes place as the lungs discharge the waste carbon dioxide from the body. They filter impurities and clear other particles that have managed to get in. There is also a role in regulating pH balance. The large intestine eliminates waste through the rectum and anus, following digestion of our food, and the skin, considered the largest organ in the body, has a role in eliminating through sweat, although it is not considered to be the major yin or yang metal organ. Excess or imbalanced metal energy can lead to many skin conditions, as well as lung and large intestine issues. The problem of "letting go" is one of the negative emotional issues associated with metal energy, as well as grieving, sadness, and even depression. So considering the metal in your chart and balancing it through the practices and five-element nutrition could have major positive effects.

METAL ELEMENT AND ORGAN FOOD TABLES

See the Fire Element and Organ Food Tables section on page 95 to review how to use the temperature column for elemental and organ balance.

Remember also that metal organs can benefit from sour foods (wood's flavor) as metal controls wood, but too much can be overwhelming. Metal organs can also benefit from sweet foods (earth's flavor), as metal is nourished by earth. Metal is weakened by water, so too many salty foods are not good for weak metal organs, but good to calm down excessive metal energy. Fire controls metal, so eating too many bitter foods can put adverse control on the metal organs. But it all depends on quantity! Whatever your required balance for harmony in your own elements, remember to eat all the five elements and colors every day!

TABLE 6.1. FOODS THAT SUPPORT METAL ORGANS AND HEALTH

FOOD	FLAVOR(S)	TEMPERATURE	YIN ORGAN	YANG ORGAN
Aniseed	Pungent, sweet	Warm	Lungs	
Apple	Sweet, sour	Cool	Lungs	
Avocado	Sweet	Cool	Lungs	Large intestine
Cauliflower	Sour	Cool		Large intestine
Cayenne	Pungent	Hot	Lungs	
Cinnamon (bark)	Pungent, bitter	Hot	Lungs	
Cinnamon (twig)	Sweet, pungent	Warm	Lungs	
Cranberry	Sweet, sour	Cold		Large intestine
Garlic	Sweet, pungent, salty	Hot	Lungs	Large intestine
Ginger (fresh)	Pungent	Hot	Lungs	Large intestine
Horseradish	Pungent	Hot	Lungs	
Leek	Pungent	Warm	Lungs	
Milk (cow or goat)	Sweet	Cool	Lungs	
Mint	Sweet, pungent	Cool	Lungs	

TABLE 6.1. FOODS THAT SUPPORT
METAL ORGANS AND HEALTH (cont.)

FOOD	FLAVOR(S)	TEMPERATURE	YIN ORGAN	YANG ORGAN
Mustard greens	Pungent	Cool	Lungs	
Nutmeg	Pungent	Warm		Large intestine
Onion (white and red)	Pungent	Warm	Lungs	
Oregano	Sweet, pungent, bitter	Warm	Lungs	
Radish	Pungent, sweet	Cool	lungs	
Scallion	Pungent, bitter	Warm	Lungs	Large intestine
Spinach	Sweet	Cool		Large intestine
Watercress	Pungent, bitter	Warm	Lungs	Large intestine

TABLE 6.2. LUNG FOODS

FOOD	FLAVOR(S)	TEMPERATURE
Almond	Sweet	Neutral
Amaranth	Sweet, bitter	Cool
Aniseed	Sweet, pungent	Warm
Apple	Sweet, sour	Cool
Apricot	Sweet, sour	Neutral
Avocado	Sweet	Cool
Bamboo shoot	Sweet	Cold
Banana	Sweet	Cold
Basil	Sweet, pungent, bitter	Warm
Cantaloupe	Sweet	Cold
Cardamom	Sweet, pungent, bitter	Warm
Carrot	Sweet	Neutral

TABLE 6.2. LUNG FOODS (cont.)

FOOD	FLAVOR(S)	TEMPERATURE
Cayenne	Pungent	Hot
Chamomile	Sweet, bitter	Cool
Cheese	Sweet, sour	Neutral
Chrysanthemum	Sweet, bitter	Cool
Cinnamon (bark)	Pungent, bitter	Hot
Cinnamon (twig)	Sweet, pungent	Warm
Coriander	Pungent	Warm
Date	Sweet	Warm
Fungus (white)	Sweet	Neutral
Garlic	Sweet, pungent, salty	Hot
Ginger (dry)	Pungent	Hot
Ginger (fresh)	Pungent	Warm
Ginseng (American)	Sweet, bitter	Neutral
Ginseng (Chinese)	Sweet	Warm
Glutinous rice (sweet rice)	Sweet	Warm
Herring	Sweet	Neutral
Honey	Sweet	Neutral
Horseradish	Pungent	Hot
Kale	Sweet, bitter	Warm
Kumquat	Pungent, sweet	Warm
Leek	Pungent	Warm
Lemon balm	Pungent, sour	Cool
Licorice	Sweet	Neutral
Lima bean	Sweet	Cool
Mandarin orange	Sweet, sour	Cold
Marjoram	Sweet, pungent	Cool

TABLE 6.2. LUNG FOODS (cont.)

FOOD	FLAVOR(S)	TEMPERATURE
Mulberry	Sweet	Cold
Mushroom (button)	Sweet	Cool
Mustard seed	Pungent	Hot
Nori (dry seaweed)	Sweet, salty	Neutral
Olive	Sweet, sour	Neutral
Onion	Pungent	Warm
Oregano	Sweet, pungent	Warm
Papaya	Sweet, bitter	Neutral
Parsnip	Sweet, pungent	Warm
Peanut (nut and oil)	Sweet	Neutral
Pear	Sweet, sour	Cool
Peppermint	Sweet, pungent	Cool
Persimmon	Sweet	Cold
Pine nut	Sweet	Warm
Pollen	Sweet, pungent, salty, sour, bitter	Neutral
Pumpkin	Sweet	Neutral
Radish	Sweet, pungent	Cool
Rosemary	Sweet, pungent	Warm
Sage	Pungent	Warm
Savory	Sweet, pungent, bitter	Warm
Scallion	Pungent, bitter	Warm
Sorghum	Sweet	Warm
Strawberry	Sweet, sour	Cool
Swiss chard	Sweet	Cool
Tangerine	Sweet, sour	Cool
Thyme	Pungent, bitter	Warm

TABLE 6.2. LUNG FOODS (cont.)

FOOD	FLAVOR(S)	TEMPERATURE
Walnut	Sweet	Warm
Water chestnut	Sweet	Cold
Watercress	Pungent, bitter	Warm

TABLE 6.3. LARGE INTESTINE FOODS

FOOD	FLAVOR(S)	TEMPERATURE
Avocado	Sweet	Cool
Banana	Sweet	Cold
Beef	Sweet	Neutral
Buckwheat	Sweet	Cool
Chamomile	Sweet, bitter	Cool
Cranberry	Sweet, sour	Cold
Cucumber	Sweet	Cool
Eggplant	Sweet	Cool
Flax	Sweet	Neutral
Fungus (black)	Sweet	Neutral
Honey	Sweet	Neutral
Kuzu	Sweet	Cool
Lemon/lime	Sour	Cold
Licorice	Sweet	Neutral
Mung bean sprout	Sweet	Cold
Mushroom (button)	Sweet	Cool
Nutmeg	Pungent	Warm
Peach	Sweet, sour	Warm
Peanut oil	Sweet	Neutral
Pepper (black)	Sweet, pungent	Hot

TABLE 6.3. LARGE INTESTINE FOODS (cont.)

FOOD	FLAVOR(S)	TEMPERATURE
Pepper (white)	Pungent, bitter	Hot
Persimmon	Sweet	Cold
Pine nut	Sweet	Warm
Plantain	Sweet	Cold
Pollen	Sweet, pungent, salty, sour, bitter	Neutral
Pumpkin seed	Sweet, bitter	Neutral
Purslane	Sour	Cold
Rhubarb	Bitter	Cold
Rose hip	Salty, sour	Neutral
Salt	Salty	Cold
Scallion	Pungent, bitter	Warm
Sorghum	Sweet	Warm
Spinach	Sweet	Cool
Swiss chard	Sweet	Cool
Tamarind	Sweet, sour	Cool
Taro root	Sweet, pungent	Neutral
Watercress	Pungent, bitter	Warm
Wheat bran	Sweet	Cool

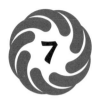

Water Element

The water element rules the kidneys and bladder, as well as the bones and the sense organs of the ears. Water energy is flexible, adaptable, and flows; it knows how to go around material and immaterial obstacles. It is the creative power of the kidneys, the yin water organ, with willpower, purpose, good feeling, peace, clear ideas, and sense of purpose. The kidneys build up the bone marrow to give the body vitality and construct the inner power of our being, our life force. The yang water organ, the bladder, stores bodily fluids for elimination and can also store chi generated through meditation. As we mentioned earlier, material energy can change into immaterial energy and vice versa. Any time you need certain types of power, you turn to your organs, and they will give you that power.

QUALITIES OF WATER

Water energy is the energy of reproduction and sexuality. When the Taoist art of geomancy, feng shui ("wind and water" is the translation), developed in ancient China, a large part of the calculations considered how water affects people—their health, wealth, relationships, family, and longevity. Studying both the still and the moving water of the rivers, streams, waterfalls, ponds, oceans, and swimming pools, and the practice of placing fish tanks in Chinese restaurants is still a vital part of feng shui today. But we also study roads, motorways, crowd movements, and other things that create flow as a form of moving water, referred to as virtual water. As traffic cannot easily turn on a ninety-degree angle, this gives us many curves in our roadways that mimic the patterns of natural waterways.

Yin water is soft, gentle moisture, like rain or dew. It is peaceful, calm, diligent, hard working, deep thinking, imaginative, adaptable, clean, honest, down-to-earth, steady, intuitive, philosophical, likable, creative, and a good teacher, lecturer, or communicator. Yin water day masters do not sit still for long. They can be cool, clearheaded, sensitive to others' feelings but often cannot manage their own feelings very well, tending to keep things private and be introverted. They commonly harbor fantasies or romantic thoughts. They value principles and can see the greater good. They are led by their hearts when pursuing careers or dreams. They can have poor staying power, can be easily distracted, and need grounding (earth phase energy) to focus on the task at hand. Water's negative emotions can make a person nervous, fearful, or even phobic.

Yang water traits are stronger and less subtle than yin water's. These people are like an ocean, lake, river, whitewater, or turbulent seas. They are intelligent, clean, adaptable, gentle, softhearted, enthusiastic, likable, extroverted, rebellious, good communicators, forceful, intuitive, persevering, sociable, noticeable, determined, resourceful, impatient, and always on the move with great, sometimes violent energy. They love adventure and physical activity; they flow around obstacles, neglecting comfort, grasping at the right opportunities and showing little signs of worry as they surf toward their goal. Their fluid path can lead to many distractions from the task at hand, as they can lose focus on their goal, distracted by the "passing ships." They are philosophical and freedom loving and uncomfortable when restrained. Comfortable grounding is important for them. Fear can sabotage the best water plans.

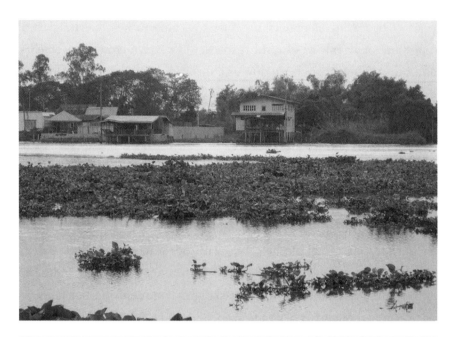

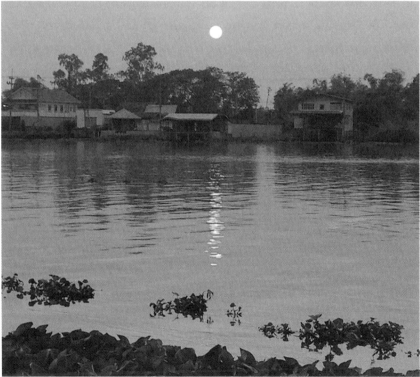

Fig. 7.1. Sunrise and sunset on the water

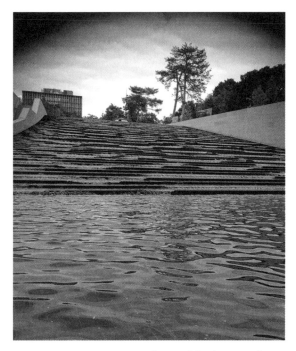

Fig. 7.2. Water cascades and finds its path.

WATER NUTRITION:
TASTE, SEASON, AND COLOR

Salt is the taste associated with the water element, but this does not mean that salt is always good for the kidneys and bladder, although it can bring on thirst, and water is essential to flushing out toxins in the urine and also stools. Let's remind ourselves that the five elements that are stored in the different organs have both their positive and negative qualities. The positive emotions associated with water are gentleness, calmness, peacefulness, and willpower, while the negative emotions associated with this element are fear and phobias. Cold is not good for the kidneys, so this region of the body should be warmly covered, especially in cold climates. Weak kidneys should also be fed with warm or hot temperature food. Salty flavor has a grounding effect as well as a softening effect, which is needed in the water season of winter. All fish that can be considered salty support water organs, as can seaweed.

Water is the gathering and flowing energy of winter and the northerly direction. Eat more sautéed food and soups in the winter to strengthen the kidneys and the bladder. Also eating foods with a warm or hot temperature and heavy foods such as grains and beans can be useful to balance out the cold of the weather.

Water's colors are black and dark blue, as seen in water foods such as seaweeds, black beans, blackberries, and black currants.

WATER SUPERFOODS

Oily fish such as mackerel, anchovies, sardines, and wild (not farmed) salmon are rich in omega-3s, a fat that is essential for making connections in the brain. These fish are good for memory, skin, and the immune system.

Seaweeds are the richest plants on our planet in terms of nutrients, minerals, and trace elements. They have been harvested and eaten fresh or preserved by drying ever since humankind first started to harvest food. Their detox properties protect us from the poisons that polluters pour into the sea, which then make their way into the food chain. Seaweeds contain fucoidan, which prevents cancer, and also vitamin levels that vary according to the variety and source of the seaweed. Their properties boost kidney energy and can prevent goiter and other thyroid issues, some cancers (notably leukemia), and also glaucoma. Seaweed reduces internal body heat and high blood pressure and disperses congestion, helping coughs. Seaweed also disperses fat concentrations in the body.

NUTRITION TO BALANCE WATER IN YOUR CHART

Begin by looking at how you can balance your water by noticing your own percentage of the element and adjusting your diet accordingly, using both the water food tables below and the water nutrition information above. Then use your knowledge of the family and phase cycles to note what will strengthen weak water or balance out excessive water.

Weak Water

Notice both if your water percentage is low and if the elements that weaken it are overly strong in your chart. If water is weak for either reason you can strengthen it by adding additional water and salty foods to your diet, and drinking more pure and healthy water. This will be even more important if both water and metal are weak, as metal is the parent of water and the element that feeds it. You will also want to notice if wood is particularly strong in your chart, as water feeds wood and can therefore be depleted by it. If you have an excess of metal in your chart, you may not need to focus as much on increasing water foods, because metal feeds water.

Excessive Water

If you have an excess of water in your chart, you may want to strengthen water's child, wood, creating balance through the family structure of the elements. The same is true for fire, water's grandchild, which can also drain water. This will be particularly true if both metal *and* water are strong in your chart. You can combat excess by lessening the water (and potentially metal) foods you are eating, but you can also create more balance by following some of the nutrition and food suggestions in the wood and fire chapters.

In addition to the dangers of excess salt for water's own organs, an excess of salty flavor can also injure the heart, cause high blood pressure and weak bones, and cause tears to fall more readily. It can be balanced by a moderate amount of sweet, earthy food.

Notice how the nutrition suggestions relate to all five elements, reminding us how important balance between all aspects of our being is. There is so much conflict in the world that we can contribute positively to its elimination by harmonizing the conflicts within ourselves.

Yin and Yang Water Organs

Look at the explanation on page 94 in the fire chapter and use the same formula to determine whether the yin (kidneys) and yang (bladder) water organs are deficient or excessive.

As we have seen, fear is associated with imbalanced water energy, and this can extend to the point of phobias. Phobias and fear can have an effect on choosing foods and how and where to eat them. So carefully considering the water in your basic natal chart could give you clues on your present choices and perhaps lead you to overcoming illogical choices.

WATER ELEMENT AND ORGAN FOOD TABLES

See the Fire Element and Organ Food Tables section on page 95 to review how to use the temperature column for elemental and organ balance.

Remember also that water organs can benefit from bitter foods (fire's flavor) as water controls fire, but too much can be overwhelming. Water organs can also benefit from pungent foods (metal's flavor), as water is nourished by metal. Water is weakened by wood, so too many sour foods are not good for weak water organs, but good to calm down excessive water energy. Earth controls water, so eating too many sweet foods can put adverse control on the earth organs. But it all depends on quantity! Whatever your required balance for harmony in your own elements, remember to eat all the five elements and colors every day!

TABLE 7.1. FOODS THAT SUPPORT
WATER ORGANS AND HEALTH

FOOD	FLAVOR(S)	TEMPERATURE	YIN ORGAN	YANG ORGAN
Anchovy (fresh)	Sweet	Warm	Kidneys	Bladder
Black bean	Sweet	Warm	Kidneys	
Black currants	Sweet, sour	Warm	Kidneys	
Cabbage	Sweet	Cool	Kidneys	
Clove	Pungent	Warm	Kidneys	
Elderflower	Sweet, pungent, bitter	Cool		Bladder
Kelp	Salty	Cool	Kidneys	
Kidney bean	Sweet	Neutral	Kidneys	Bladder
Lentil	Sweet	Neutral	Kidneys	Bladder
Mackerel (fresh)	Sweet	Neutral	Kidneys	Bladder
Millet	Sweet, salty	Cool	Kidneys	
Nettle	Sweet, salty	Cool	Kidneys	Bladder
Oats	Sweet	Warm	Kidneys	
Parsley	Pungent, sweet, salty	Warm		Bladder
Pork	Sweet, salty	Neutral	Kidneys	
Quinoa	Sweet, sour	Warm	Kidneys	
Rice (wild)	Sweet, sour	Cool	Kidneys	Bladder
Salmon (fresh, wild)	Sweet	Neutral	Kidneys	Bladder
Sardine	Sweet, salty	Neutral	Kidneys	Bladder
Seaweed (general)	Salty	Cold	Kidneys	
Sweet potato and yam	Sweet	Cool	Kidneys	
Trout	Sweet, salty	Warm	Kidneys	

TABLE 7.2. KIDNEY FOODS

FOOD	FLAVOR(S)	TEMPERATURE
Adzuki bean	Sweet, sour	Neutral
Aloe vera	Bitter	Neutral
Asparagus	Sweet, bitter	Cold
Black currant	Sweet, sour	Cool
Celery	Sweet, bitter	Cool
Clam (freshwater)	Sweet, salty	Cold
Cranberry	Sweet, sour	Cold
Cuttlefish	Salty	Neutral
Duck	Sweet	Neutral
Fava bean	Sweet	Neutral
Ginseng (American)	Sweet, bitter	Neutral
Grape	Sweet, sour	Neutral
Kidney bean	Sweet	Neutral
Lemon/lime	Sour	Cold
Lentil	Sweet	Neutral
Licorice	Sweet	Neutral
Marjoram	Sweet, pungent	Cool
Millet	Sweet, salty	Cool
Mulberry	Sweet	Cold
Nettle	Sweet, salty	Cool
Pistachio	Sweet, sour, bitter	Neutral
Salt	Salty	Cold
Seaweed	Salty	Cold
Spinach	Sweet	Cool
Strawberry	Sweet, sour	Cool
Wild Rice	Sweet, sour	Cool

TABLE 7.3. BLADDER FOODS

FOOD	FLAVOR(S)	TEMPERATURE
Elderflower	Sweet, pungent, bitter	Cool
Licorice	Sweet	Neutral
Nettle	Sweet, salty	Cool
Parsley	Pungent, salty, bitter	Warm
Pollen	Sweet, pungent, salty, sour, bitter	Neutral
Pomegranate	Sweet, sour	Neutral
Purslane	Sour	Cold
Rose hip	Salty, sour	Neutral
Watermelon	Sweet	Cold
Wax gourd (or winter gourd or winter melon)	Sweet	Cool
Wild rice	Sweet, sour	Cool

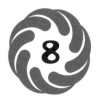

Wood Element

Wood rules the liver, the yin wood organ, and the gallbladder, the yang wood organ, as well as the tendons, the muscles, and the sense organs of the eyes. Wood energy is the big-picture thinker and takes this kind of thinking forward into speculation; its organizational gifts are that of the visionary rather than the earth's socially oriented management of people.

THE QUALITIES OF WOOD

The wood organs, the liver and gallbladder, store the virtues of generosity and kindness and the negative emotions of anger and jealousy. The liver is about control—it must control the tendons and ligaments to keep the body in place and moving well, supple and flexible. The liver can be compared to a general or commander in chief of the armed forces, who must know when to remain firm and when to use flexibility and bend with the situation. The liver must assess circumstances, from which stems its conception and planning skills. The gallbladder stores the bile produced in the liver, although it is fairly full of bile and can store less chi than the bladder does.

Wood's negative energies are the flammable ones of anger and jealousy. Just as a general brought to anger will lose his ability to follow his own strategy and command properly, wood's emotions can fuel fire's

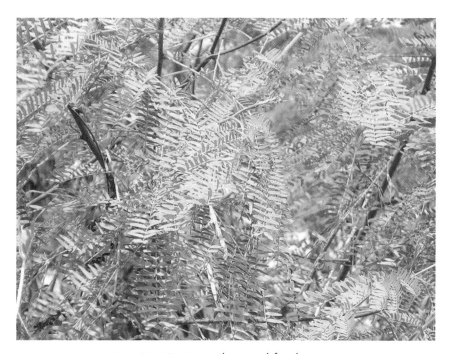

Fig. 8.1. Can't see the wood for the trees

outbursts because wood feeds fire; wood can weaken itself by burning up in this way. Wood people's stress must be managed to enable proper use of all of their talents. Many people with strong wood feel that they must have a lot of fire, as they get excited and even angry easily, which they think must be fiery. But in fact it is because they have an excess of wood to throw on the flames, so it is less about the passion of fire and more about the anger of wood.

Wood is a very creative energy, the energy of spring and the beginning of growth and creation: art and all forms of writing are gifts common to strong wood-energy people. Accordingly, the love of literature, writing, and publishing are considered wood aspects, as are learning and education. Good teachers and good students will have significant wood energy, as they can use wood's creativity combined with the planning and vision of teaching curricula. In an astrological chart it is considered quite lucky to have wood as an incoming energy

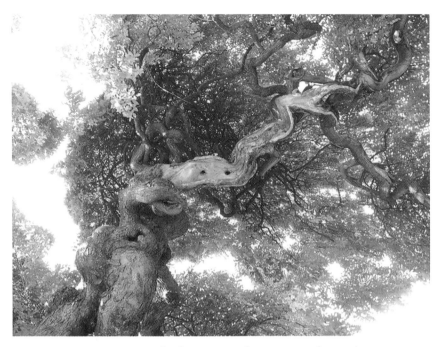

Fig. 8.2. Wood—the energy of creation and growth

during one's school and university years, if it is not too excessive, as learning will become a focus, making it easier for the person to study, whatever his or her level and abilities. The choices made for school and university subjects often reflect the ten-year cycle energy of that time as well as the natal chart.

The planning and strategy skills of wood people mean that it is a typical energy used by lawyers and even salesmen. The connection with actual wood itself and plants means that it is usually a strong element in gardeners and garden designers, herbalists, naturopaths, or anyone using the power of plants and wood-related industries that involve paper, such as writing and publishing. It is the forward planning and visionary design of an architect.

Yang wood is the energy of the large tree: strong and unbending, powerful, steady, forthright, direct, stern, down-to-earth, straightforward, sturdy, stubborn, reliable, supportive, outspoken, determined, and righteous. Planning and vision are its strong points, together with an ability to see a project through to the end, like a tree reaching upward toward sunlight. It is an honorable energy, reaching for the clear sky and heavens. It is deep rooted, serious, and professional, with a keen sense of responsibility. Those with dominant yang wood exhibit strong willpower and do not give up easily in the face of adversity; their reputation and morals are an important issue for them. They are sympathetic to those in need of help but can be authoritarian, bossy, predictable, slow witted, and slow to change or compromise. They can be stiff and thick skinned when it comes to understanding what is happening around them, giving the impression that they are uncaring. Those with dominant yin wood are like flowers and plants—soft, meek, and mild, but flexible, adaptable, fickle, expressive, extroverted, charismatic, creative, manipulative, quick witted, possessive, careful, and good with money. Yin wood day masters are survivors, good motivators, and good project leaders. Yin wood also reaches upward, finding its way in life like the winding shoots that eventually reach the sunlight at the top of the forest canopy. Fragile-looking strands of yin wood vines and creepers can be platted together to make tough string and rope. Yin wood day masters know how to skirt around trouble but can be timid and easily swayed and change their minds and strategy easily according to circumstances. With a tendency to hold grudges, they may be easily deceived or misled, give way to temptation or lose confidence quickly, but if well rooted, they can survive a storm easier than yang wood.

WOOD NUTRITION:
TASTE, SEASON, AND COLOR

Sour, the taste of wood foods, includes many leafy vegetables, acidic fruits and their juices, and vinegars. An excess or lack of sour food can weaken the wood organs of the liver and gallbladder. Sour foods such as lemons and limes can draw energy inward, to be used wherever there is abnormal fluid leakage or prolapsed organs. The sour flavor can also balance an excess of sweet flavor and have a gathering effect required in wood's spring season.

Wood is the growth of the springtime, the energy of rising sap in plants and trees. You can eat more steamed food during the spring to strengthen the liver and gallbladder. At this time it's also important to *eat your greens!* Wood is the green season and the green color, along with light blue and turquoise, and of course, wood foods include green vegetables. Add liberal amounts of green vegetables to your diet from a wide range of sources. Chlorophyll, a green pigment found in plants and grasses, is plant "blood" and is very cleansing for the wood organs. Green foods such as wheatgrass and barley grass are some of the lowest calorific or sugar-rich foods on the planet and the most nutritious. Something green in the morning is a good way to "break the fast" as it is good for the liver. This is when your digestive juices are strong, so you should be sure to have a good breakfast. In China, as in many other countries, it's traditional to eat a good breakfast with five element overtures to the day, including green foods and usually some sour-tasting ones too. However, in the West breakfast is mainly earth and metal and the colors white and yellow—eggs, cereal, milk, yogurt, white bread—meaning that all of the five elements are not represented or eaten.

WOOD SUPERFOODS

Apples ("An apple a day keeps the doctor away") are very high in antioxidants and reduce the risk of asthma, cancer, diabetes, and cardiovascular disease.

Bergamot is a relative of the lemon and can easily be substituted for lemon in cooking; it can also be used as a juice or an extract. It has many of the lemon's properties, plus unique flavonoids. The taste is less acid and more orangey; it is used as a distinctive hint of flavor in Earl Grey tea and is extensively used in the perfume industry. Its many health-giving properties make it worthy of superfood status. Buy only organic, wash well, and also use the zest and pith.

Broccoli is known as helpful in preventing cancers (breast, uterus, lung, liver, kidneys, etc.) and is also known for its detoxifying properties. It is a rich source of vitamin C, fiber, amino acids, and sulfur. Its nutrients are good for the eyes, bones, and immune system and for stomach disorders.

Coconut is an amazing superfood that contains copper, fiber, selenium, and vitamin C. Its properties help the bones, blood sugar, weight loss, joint inflammation, and arthritis, and it promotes youthful skin. The selenium facilitates mind and body relaxation. Coconut oil has become highly recommended by modern nutritionists despite containing saturated fats. Indeed, Pacific Island populations that have traditionally cooked with it are virtually free of heart diseases and colon cancer, arteriosclerosis, kidney disease, and high cholesterol. Coconut water is cooling to the stomach, so can help digestion problems. Coconut oil is one of the good fats to use in cooking, as it is a fat that the body can easily convert into energy.

Kale helps prevent skin diseases and has anti-inflammatory and anti-cancer properties. It also facilitates liver detox. To eat it raw in a salad, wash well, remove and throw away the central spine, cut up the rest of the leaves, dry them off, and then with the hands lightly massage a healthy oil dressing into the pieces of leaves rather than tossing it over the kale. In this way the oil breaks the surface tension of the leaves, coating them, and the kale does not taste quite so bitter.

Mulberries are traditionally known in Asia for being good for blood circulation, diabetes, dizziness, insomnia, constipation, fever, infections, eyes, internal organs, joints, and even depression. Mulberries are coming back into fashion, as their many healthful compounds are widely recognized. In health food stores they can be found in organic biscuits and cereal bars and are also believed to help prevent cancer.

Pomegranates are a generous source of antimicrobial and antioxidant compounds that flush out harmful toxins, resulting in a slimmer body and shiny skin. Their properties help prevent cancer and regulate blood pressure. They are effective against dental plaque and bad cholesterol and possibly prevent the onset of Alzheimer's disease and osteoarthritis. They can also improve erectile function in men and are good for heart function.

NUTRITION TO BALANCE WOOD IN YOUR CHART

Look at your wood percentage in your five-element chart and determine whether it seems weak or strong. Then notice its relationship to the other elements based on the family and phase models. Use the wood nutrition information above and below and the food tables to help adjust your diet in a way that will bring more overall balance to your system.

Weak Wood

As we have learned, wood can be weak in comparison to the other percentages on your chart, but it can also be weakened by its relationship to the other elements. If your wood is weak or is greatly weakened by the elements around it, you can strengthen it by adding more wood foods to your diet.

If your fire element is quite strong, you may want to add even more wood into your diet, as wood feeds fire and may be depleted by an excess of that element. If you have a lot of water in your chart, you may not need to focus as much on increasing wood foods, even if wood is fairly weak, because water is the parent and feeder of wood.

Excessive Wood

If you have a large percentage of wood in your chart, you may want to strengthen wood's child, fire, so that it can absorb some of wood's energy. You could also strengthen the element that wood controls, earth, which is wood's grandchild and therefore also absorbs energy from wood. If both water *and* wood are strong in your chart, this will be even more important for balance. You can use the nutrition suggestions and food tables in the fire and earth chapters to help achieve this balance.

In addition to damaging the wood organs, the liver and gallbladder, an excess of sour flavor can also injure the spleen and stomach, the earth organs. This can be balanced by pungent foods—the flavor of metal.

Making sure all of the tastes, colors, and elements are represented on your plate and noting which proportions will help bring the most balance to your individual five-element makeup will help create vitality and well-being physically, emotionally, mentally, and spiritually.

Yin and Yang Wood Organs

Look at the explanation on page 94 in the fire chapter, and use the same formula to determine whether the yin (liver) and yang (gallbladder) wood organs are deficient or excessive.

Even with high wood energy in your chart, you should not neglect to eat something green every day. The liver works super hard; it is the real chemical production plant of the body, and even if it has high energy, it still needs to keep going around the clock. That is why total fasting must be very carefully supervised, as a complete absence of food intake will give the liver too much opportunity to produce bile to stock in the gallbladder, which will not have an opportunity to off-load it during digestion (if there is nothing at all going in). You can read more about this in the authors' *Pi Gu Chi Kung: Inner Alchemy Energy Fasting*.

WOOD ELEMENT AND ORGAN FOOD TABLES

See the Fire Element and Organ Food Tables section on page 95 to review how to use the temperature column for element and organ balance.

Remember also that wood organs can benefit from sweet foods (earth's flavor), as wood controls earth, but too much can be overwhelming. Wood organs can also benefit from salty foods (water's flavor), as wood is nourished by water. Wood is weakened by fire, so too many bitter foods are not good for weak wood organs, but good to calm down excessive wood energy. Metal controls wood, so eating too many pungent foods can put adverse control on the wood organs. But it all depends on quantity! Whatever your required balance for harmony in your own elements, remember to eat all the five elements and colors every day!

TABLE 8.1. FOODS THAT SUPPORT WOOD ORGANS AND HEALTH

FOOD	FLAVOR(S)	TEMPERATURE	YIN ORGAN	YANG ORGAN
Adzuki bean	Sweet, sour	Neutral	Liver	
Apple	Sweet, sour	Cool		Gallbladder
Avocado	Sweet	Cool	Liver	
Beet	Sweet	Neutral	Liver	
Bergamot	Sour	Warm	Liver	Gallbladder
Bok choy	Pungent	Cool	Liver	Gallbladder
Broccoli	Pungent, bitter	Cool	Liver	Gallbladder
Cabbage (green, spring)	Sour, bitter	Neutral	Liver	Gallbladder
Chinese cabbage	Sweet, pungent	Neutral	Liver	Gallbladder
Chive	Pungent	Warm	Liver	
Kale	Sweet, bitter	Warm	Liver	Gallbladder
Kelp	Salty	Cold	Liver	
Lemon	Sour	Cold	Liver	Gallbladder
Lettuce	Sweet, bitter	Cool	Liver	Gallbladder
Lime	Sour	Cold	Liver	Gallbladder
Mulberry	Sweet	Cold	Liver	

TABLE 8.1. FOODS THAT SUPPORT
WOOD ORGANS AND HEALTH (cont.)

FOOD	FLAVOR(S)	TEMPERATURE	YIN ORGAN	YANG ORGAN
Pineapple	Sweet, sour	Hot	Liver	
Plum	Sweet, sour	Neutral	Liver	
Raspberry	Sweet, sour	Neutral	Liver	
Rye	Bitter	Neutral	Liver	Gallbladder
Sesame seed	Sweet	Neutral	Liver	
Spinach	Sweet, pungent	Cool	Liver	Gallbladder
Swiss chard	Sweet, pungent	Cool	Liver	Gallbladder

TABLE 8.2. LIVER FOODS

FOOD	FLAVOR(S)	TEMPERATURE
Adzuki bean	Sweet, sour	Neutral
Artichoke	Sweet, salty, bitter	Cool
Avocado	Sweet	Cool
Blackberry	Sweet, sour	Warm
Black currant	Sweet, sour	Cool
Carrot	Sweet	Neutral
Celery	Sweet, bitter	Cool
Chamomile	Sweet, bitter	Cool
Chinese chive	Pungent	Warm
Chrysanthemum	Sweet, bitter	Cool
Clam (freshwater)	Sweet, salty	Cold
Crab	Salty	Cold
Cumin	Pungent	Warm
Dandelion (leaf and root)	Sweet, salty, bitter	Cold

TABLE 8.2. LIVER FOODS (cont.)

FOOD	FLAVOR(S)	TEMPERATURE
Dongui	Sweet, pungent	Warm
Eggplant	Sweet	Cool
Elderflower	Sweet, pungent, bitter	Cool
Fenugreek seed	Bitter	Warm
Flax	Sweet	Neutral
Fungus (white)	Sweet	Neutral
Garlic	Sweet, pungent, salty	Hot
Grape	Sweet, sour	Neutral
Hawthorn	Sweet, sour	Warm
Jasmine	Sweet, pungent	Warm
Kumquat	Pungent, sweet	Warm
Leek	Pungent	Warm
Lemon balm	Pungent, sour	Cool
Lemon/lime	Sour	Cold
Licorice	Sweet	Neutral
Lima bean	Sweet	Cool
Linseed	Sweet	Neutral
Liver (beef)	Sweet	Neutral
Liver (chicken)	Sweet	Warm
Mackerel	Sweet	Neutral
Mulberry	Sweet	Cold
Mussel	Salty	Warm
Nettle	Sweet, salty	Cool
Olive oil	Sweet	Neutral
Peppermint	Sweet, pungent	Cool
Pineapple	Sweet, sour	Hot

TABLE 8.2. LIVER FOODS (cont.)

FOOD	FLAVOR(S)	TEMPERATURE
Pine nut	Sweet	Warm
Pistachio	Sweet, sour, bitter	Neutral
Pollen	Sweet, pungent, salty, sour, bitter	Neutral
Purslane	Sour	Cold
Radish	Sweet, pungent	Cool
Raspberry	Sweet, sour	Neutral
Rosemary	Sweet, pungent	Warm
Rye	Bitter	Neutral
Saffron	Pungent	Neutral
Sesame (black)	Sweet	Neutral
Shrimp or prawn	Sweet	Warm
Squash (butternut, spaghetti)	Sweet, sour	Warm
Star anise	Sweet, pungent	Warm
Strawberry	Sweet, sour	Cool
Tomato	Sweet, sour	Cold
Vinegar	Sour, bitter	Warm

TABLE 8.3. GALLBLADDER FOODS

FOOD	FLAVOR(S)	TEMPERATURE
Artichoke	Sweet, salty, bitter	Cool
Dandelion (leaf and root)	Sweet, salty, bitter	Cold
Lemon/lime	Sour	Cold
Licorice	Sweet	Neutral
Pollen	Sweet, pungent, salty, sour, bitter	Neutral
Rye	Bitter	Neutral

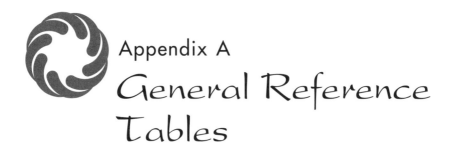

Appendix A
General Reference Tables

TABLE A.1.
ELEMENTS, ORGANS,
EMOTIONS, AND HEALING SOUNDS

ELEMENT	YIN ORGAN(S)	YANG ORGAN	POSITIVE EMOTIONS	NEGATIVE EMOTIONS	HEALING SOUNDS
FIRE	Heart	Small intestine	Love, joy, compassion	Hatred, cruelty, impatience, arrogance	Haw-w-w-w-w-w
EARTH	Spleen, pancreas	Stomach	Fairness, openness, trust	Worry, anxiety	Who-oo-oo-oo
METAL	Lungs	Large intestine	Motivation, courage, righteousness	Depression, sadness, grief	Sss-s-s-s-s-s
WATER	Kidneys	Bladder	Willpower, gentleness, fluidity	Fear and phobias	Choo-oo-oo-oo
WOOD	Liver	Gallbladder	Kindness, generosity	Anger, jealousy, stress	Sh-h-h-h-h-h

TABLE A.2.
ELEMENTS, SEASONS,
FLAVORS, COLORS, AND ORGANS

ELEMENT	SEASON	FLAVOR(S)/ TASTE(S)	COLOR(S)	YIN ORGAN(S)	YANG ORGAN
FIRE	Summer	Bitter	Red, purple, pink	Heart	Small intestine
EARTH	All "in between" seasons, such as "Indian" summer	Sweet	Yellow, beige, brown	Spleen, pancreas	Stomach
METAL	Autumn	Pungent, hot	White, gold, silver, bronze	Lungs	Large intestine
WATER	Winter	Salty	Black, dark blue	Kidneys	Bladder
WOOD	Spring	Sour	Green, light blue, turquoise	Liver	Gallbladder

TABLE A.3.
FAMILY AND PHASE* OF ELEMENTS

ELEMENT	SIBLING / SELF	PARENT / RESOURCE	CHILD / EXPRESSION	GRANDCHILD / WEALTH	GRANDPARENT / POWER
FIRE	Fire	Wood	Earth	Metal	Water
EARTH	Earth	Fire	Metal	Water	Wood
METAL	Metal	Earth	Water	Wood	Fire
WATER	Water	Metal	Wood	Fire	Earth
WOOD	Wood	Water	Fire	Earth	Metal

*Note that the phase is indicated in the pictogram on your natal chart.

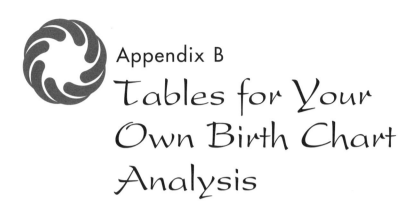

Appendix B

Tables for Your Own Birth Chart Analysis

TABLE A.4.
YOUR ELEMENTAL
RELATIONSHIPS AND PHASES

Fill in the Blank Spaces based on Your Natal Chart

ELEMENT	RELATIONSHIP	PHASE	PERCENTAGE
Day Master:	Self/Sibling	Self	
	Child	Expression	
	Grandchild	Wealth	
	Grandparent	Power	
	Parent	Resource	

TABLE A.5.

YOUR ORGAN ANALYSIS CHART

Fill in the Blank Values to Determine Your Organ Strength

ELEMENT	ORGAN	VALUE
Yin Fire	Heart	
Yang Fire	Small intestine	
Yin Earth	Spleen, pancreas	
Yang Earth	Stomach	
Yin Metal	Lungs	
Yang Metal	Large intestine	
Yin Water	Kidneys	
Yang Water	Bladder	
Yin Wood	Liver	
Yang Wood	Gallbladder	

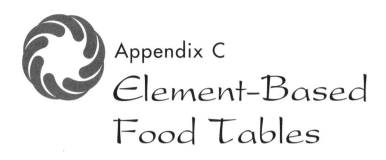

Appendix C
Element-Based Food Tables

TABLE A.6.
FOODS THAT SUPPORT
FIRE ORGANS AND HEALTH

FOOD	FLAVOR(S)	TEMPERATURE	YIN ORGAN	YANG ORGAN
Adzuki bean	Sweet, sour	Neutral	Heart	Small intestine
Aloe vera	Bitter	Neutral	Heart	
Artichoke	Sweet, salty, bitter	Cool	Heart	
Asparagus	Sweet, bitter	Cold		Small intestine
Banana	Sweet	Cold	Heart	Small intestine
Basil	Sweet, pungent, bitter	Warm	Heart	
Blueberry	Sour	Cool	Heart	
Cabbage	Sweet	Cool		Small intestine
Cauliflower	Sour	Cool	Heart	Small intestine
Cacao	Bitter, sweet	Warm	Heart	Small intestine
Chickpea	Sweet	Neutral	Heart	Small intestine
Eggplant	Sweet	Cool	Heart	
Onion	Pungent, sweet	Warm	Heart	Small intestine
Pepper (chili)	Pungent	Hot	Heart	

TABLE A.6.
FOODS THAT SUPPORT
FIRE ORGANS AND HEALTH (cont.)

FOOD	FLAVOR(S)	TEMPERATURE	YIN ORGAN	YANG ORGAN
Plum (Victoria, European, sweet, and purple)	Sweet, sour	Warm	Heart	Small intestine
Pomegranate	Sweet, sour	Neutral	Heart	
Rosemary	Sweet, pungent	Warm	Heart	
Saffron	Pungent	Neutral	Heart	
Sage	Pungent	Warm		
Scallion	Sweet, bitter	Warm	Heart	
Seaweed	Sweet, salty	Cool	Heart	Small intestine
Spinach	Sweet	Cool		Small intestine
Tomato (red)	Sweet, sour	Warm (when sweet and ripe)		Small intestine
Thyme	Pungent, bitter	Warm	Heart	
Turmeric	Pungent, bitter	Warm	Heart	

TABLE A.7. FOODS THAT SUPPORT
EARTH ORGANS AND HEALTH

FOOD	FLAVOR(S)	TEMPERATURE	YIN ORGANS	YANG ORGAN
Alfalfa seed	Bitter	Cool	Spleen, pancreas	Stomach
Alfalfa sprout	Salty, bitter	Cool	Spleen, pancreas	Stomach
Aloe vera	Bitter	Neutral	Spleen, pancreas	Stomach
Apricot	Sweet, sour	Neutral	Spleen, pancreas	
Avocado	Sweet	Cool	Spleen, pancreas	
Banana	Sweet	Cold	Spleen, pancreas	Stomach
Beef	Sweet	Neutral	Spleen, pancreas	Stomach
Black pepper	Sweet, pungent	Hot		Stomach
Blueberry	Sour	Cool	Spleen, pancreas	Stomach
Buckwheat	Sweet	Cool	Spleen, pancreas	Stomach
Carrot	Sweet	Neutral	Spleen, pancreas	
Cauliflower	Sour	Cool	Spleen, pancreas	Stomach
Celery	Sweet, bitter	Cool	Spleen, pancreas	Stomach
Cherry	Sweet	Warm	Spleen, pancreas	Stomach
Chicken	Sweet	Warm	Spleen, pancreas	Stomach
Coriander (leaf)	Pungent	Warm	Spleen, pancreas	
Cucumber	Sweet	Cool	Spleen, pancreas	Stomach

TABLE A.7. FOODS THAT SUPPORT
EARTH ORGANS AND HEALTH (cont.)

FOOD	FLAVOR(S)	TEMPERATURE	YIN ORGANS	YANG ORGAN
Eggs (chicken)	Sweet	Warm		Stomach
Fig (fresh or dried)	Sweet	Cool	Spleen, pancreas	Stomach
Garlic	Sweet, pungent, salty	Hot	Spleen, pancreas	Stomach
Grape	Sweet, sour	Warm	Spleen, pancreas	
Green bean (string bean)	Sweet	Neutral	Spleen, pancreas	Stomach
Jasmine	Sweet, pungent	Warm	Spleen, pancreas	
Kale	Sweet, bitter	Warm		Stomach
Millet	Sweet, salty	Cool	Spleen, pancreas	Stomach
Oat	Sweet	Warm	Spleen, pancreas	Stomach
Parsley	Pungent, salty, bitter	Warm		Stomach
Parsnip	Sweet, pungent	Warm	Spleen, pancreas	
Quinoa (white)	Sweet, sour	Warm		Stomach
Radish	Pungent, sweet	Cool		Stomach
Rosemary	Sweet, pungent	Warm	Spleen, pancreas	
Sesame oil	Sweet, pungent	Cool		Stomach
Sweet potato	Sweet	Neutral	Spleen, pancreas	
Tomato	Sweet, sour	Cold		Stomach
Watermelon	Sweet	Cold		Stomach

TABLE A.8. FOODS THAT SUPPORT
METAL ORGANS AND HEALTH

FOOD	FLAVOR(S)	TEMPERATURE	YIN ORGAN	YANG ORGAN
Aniseed	Pungent, sweet	Warm	Lungs	
Apple	Sweet, sour	Cool	Lungs	
Avocado	Sweet	Cool	Lungs	Large intestine
Cauliflower	Sour	Cool		Large intestine
Cayenne	Pungent	Hot	Lungs	
Cinnamon (bark)	Pungent, bitter	Hot	Lungs	
Cinnamon (twig)	Sweet, pungent	Warm	Lungs	
Cranberry	Sweet, sour	Cold		Large intestine
Garlic	Sweet, pungent, salty	Hot	Lungs	Large intestine
Ginger (fresh)	Pungent	Hot	Lungs	Large intestine
Horseradish	Pungent	Hot	Lungs	
Leek	Pungent	Warm	Lungs	
Milk (cow or goat)	Sweet	Cool	Lungs	
Mint	Sweet, pungent	Cool	Lungs	
Mustard greens	Pungent	Cool	Lungs	
Nutmeg	Pungent	Warm		Large intestine
Onion (white and red)	Pungent	Warm	Lungs	
Oregano	Sweet, pungent, bitter	Warm	Lungs	
Radish	Pungent, sweet	Cool	Lungs	
Scallion	Pungent, bitter	Warm	Lungs	Large intestine
Spinach	Sweet	Cool		Large intestine
Watercress	Pungent, bitter	Warm	Lungs	Large intestine

TABLE A.9. FOODS THAT SUPPORT
WATER ORGANS AND HEALTH

FOOD	FLAVOR(S)	TEMPERATURE	YIN ORGAN	YANG ORGAN
Anchovy (fresh)	Sweet	Warm	Kidneys	Bladder
Black bean	Sweet	Warm	Kidneys	
Black currants	Sweet, sour	Warm	Kidneys	
Cabbage	Sweet	Cool	Kidneys	
Clove	Pungent	Warm	Kidneys	
Elderflower	Sweet, pungent, bitter	Cool		Bladder
Kelp	Salty	Cool	Kidneys	
Kidney bean	Sweet	Neutral	Kidneys	Bladder
Lentil	Sweet	Neutral	Kidneys	Bladder
Mackerel (fresh)	Sweet	Neutral	Kidneys	Bladder
Millet	Sweet, salty	Cool	Kidneys	
Nettle	Sweet, salty	Cool	Kidney	Bladder
Oats	Sweet	Warm	Kidneys	
Parsley	Pungent, sweet, salty	Warm		Bladder
Pork	Sweet, salty	Neutral	Kidneys	
Quinoa	Sweet, sour	Warm	Kidneys	
Rice (wild)	Sweet, sour	Cool	Kidneys	Bladder
Salmon (fresh, wild)	Sweet	Neutral	Kidneys	Bladder
Sardine	Sweet, salty	Neutral	Kidneys	Bladder
Seaweed (general)	Salty	Cold	Kidneys	
Sweet potato and yam	Sweet	Cool	Kidneys	
Trout	Sweet, salty	Warm	Kidneys	

TABLE A.10. FOODS THAT SUPPORT
WOOD ORGANS AND HEALTH

FOOD	FLAVOR(S)	TEMPERATURE	YIN ORGAN	YANG ORGAN
Adzuki bean	Sweet, sour	Neutral	Liver	
Apple	Sweet, sour	Cool		Gallbladder
Avocado	Sweet	Cool	Liver	
Beet	Sweet	Neutral	Liver	
Bergamot	Sour	Warm	Liver	Gallbladder
Bok choy	Pungent	Cool	Liver	Gallbladder
Broccoli	Pungent, bitter	Cool	Liver	Gallbladder
Cabbage (green, spring)	Sour, bitter	Neutral	Liver	Gallbladder
Chinese cabbage	Sweet, pungent	Neutral	Liver	Gallbladder
Chive	Pungent	Warm	Liver	
Kale	Sweet, bitter	Warm	Liver	Gallbladder
Kelp	Salty	Cold	Liver	
Lemon	Sour	Cold	Liver	Gallbladder
Lettuce	Sweet, bitter	Cool	Liver	Gallbladder
Lime	Sour	Cold	Liver	Gallbladder
Mulberry	Sweet	Cold	Liver	
Pineapple	Sweet, sour	Hot	Liver	
Plum	Sweet, sour	Neutral	Liver	
Raspberry	Sweet, sour	Neutral	Liver	
Rye	Bitter	Neutral	Liver	Gallbladder
Sesame seed	Sweet	Neutral	Liver	
Spinach	Sweet, pungent	Cool	Liver	Gallbladder
Swiss chard	Sweet, pungent	Cool	Liver	Gallbladder

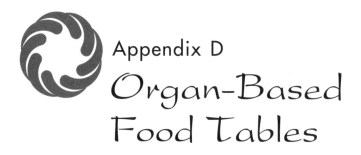

Appendix D
Organ-Based Food Tables

TABLE A.11.
HEART FOODS

FOOD	FLAVOR(S)	TEMPERATURE
Adzuki bean	Sweet, sour	Neutral
Almond	Sweet	Neutral
Aloe vera	Bitter	Neutral
Aniseed	Sweet, pungent	Warm
Apple	Sweet, sour	Cool
Cherry	Sweet	Warm
Chickpea	Sweet	Neutral
Chili	Pungent	Hot
Cinnamon (twig)	Sweet, pungent	Warm
Garlic	Sweet, pungent, salty	Hot
Hawthorn	Sweet, sour	Warm
Lentil	Sweet	Neutral
Licorice	Sweet	Neutral
Marjoram	Sweet, pungent	Cool
Mung bean	Sweet	Cool
Pepper (black)	Sweet, pungent	Hot

TABLE A.11.
HEART FOODS (cont.)

FOOD	FLAVOR(S)	TEMPERATURE
Persimmon	Sweet	Cold
Pollen	Sweet, pungent, salty, sour, bitter	Neutral
Rosemary	Sweet, pungent	Warm
Saffron	Pungent	Neutral
Scallion	Pungent, bitter	Warm
Watermelon	Sweet	Cold
Wheat germ	Pungent	Cold

TABLE A.12. SMALL INTESTINE FOODS

FOODS	FLAVOR(S)	TEMPERATURE
Adzuki bean	Sweet, sour	Neutral
Licorice	Sweet	Neutral
Mushroom (button)	Sweet	Cool
Peach	Sweet, sour	Warm
Pepper (white)	Pungent, bitter	Hot
Plantain	Sweet	Cold
Pollen	Sweet, pungent, salty, sour, bitter	Neutral
Salt	Salty	Cold
Spinach	Sweet	Cool
Tamarind	Sweet, sour	Cool
Wheat germ	Pungent	Cold

TABLE A.13. SPLEEN AND PANCREAS FOODS

FOOD	FLAVOR(S)	TEMPERATURE
Almonds	Sweet	Neutral
Aloe vera	Bitter	Neutral
Aniseed	Sweet, pungent	Warm
Avocado	Sweet	Cool
Barley	Sweet, salty	Cool
Beef	Sweet	Neutral
Buckwheat	Sweet	Cool
Caraway	Sweet, pungent	Warm
Carp	Sweet	Neutral
Carrot	Sweet	Neutral
Cayenne	Pungent	Hot
Celery	Sweet, bitter	Cool
Chamomile	Sweet, bitter	Cool
Cherry	Sweet	Warm
Chicken	Sweet	Warm
Chili	Pungent	Hot
Chinese date (red, black, jujube)	Sweet	Neutral
Cinnamon (bark)	Pungent, bitter	Hot
Clove	Pungent	Warm
Coriander (leaf)	Pungent	Warm
Cucumber	Sweet	Cool
Cumin	Pungent	Warm
Dandelion (leaf and root)	Sweet, salty, bitter	Cold
Dill seed	Pungent	Warm
Dongui	Sweet, pungent	Warm
Eggplant	Sweet	Cool
Fennel seed	Sweet, pungent	Warm

TABLE A.13. SPLEEN AND PANCREAS FOODS (cont.)

FOOD	FLAVOR(S)	TEMPERATURE
Flax	Sweet	Neutral
Garlic	Sweet, pungent, salty	Hot
Ginger (dry)	Pungent	Hot
Ginger (fresh)	Pungent	Warm
Ginseng (American)	Sweet, bitter	Neutral
Ginseng (Chinese)	Sweet	Warm
Glutinous rice (sweet rice)	Sweet	Warm
Grapes	Sweet, sour	Warm
Hawthorn	Sweet, sour	Warm
Hawthorn (berry)	Sweet, sour	Cool
Herring	Sweet	Neutral
Honey	Sweet	Neutral
Juniper	Sweet, pungent, bitter	Warm
Kumquat	Pungent, sweet	Warm
Kuzu	Sweet	Cool
Lamb	Sweet	Hot
Leek	Pungent	Warm
Lentil	Sweet	Neutral
Licorice	Sweet	Neutral
Linseed	Sweet	Neutral
Mandarin orange	Sweet, sour	Cold
Marjoram	Sweet, pungent	Cool
Millet	Sweet, salty	Cool
Mushroom (button)	Sweet	Cool
Nettle	Sweet, salty	Cool
Nutmeg	Pungent	Warm
Oat	Sweet	Warm

TABLE A.13. SPLEEN AND PANCREAS FOODS (cont.)

FOOD	FLAVOR(S)	TEMPERATURE
Papaya	Sweet, bitter	Neutral
Pea	Sweet	Cool
Peanut oil	Sweet	Neutral
Peppermint	Sweet, pungent	Cool
Persimmon	Sweet	Cold
Pollen	Sweet, pungent, salty, sour, bitter	Neutral
Pork	Sweet, salty	Neutral
Potato	Sweet	Neutral
Pumpkin	Sweet	Neutral
Pumpkin seed	Sweet, bitter	Neutral
Quince	Sour	Warm
Rice	Sweet	Neutral
Rosemary	Sweet, pungent	Warm
Rye	Bitter	Neutral
Salmon	Sweet	Neutral
Sardine	Sweet, salty	Neutral
Sorghum	Sweet	Warm
Spelt	Sweet	Warm
Squash	Sweet	Warm
Star anise	Sweet, pungent	Warm
Strawberry	Sweet, sour	Cool
Sunflower seed	Sweet	Neutral
Swiss chard	Sweet	Cool
Taro root	Sweet, pungent	Neutral
Thyme	Pungent, bitter	Warm
Watercress	Pungent, bitter	Warm

TABLE A.14. STOMACH FOODS

FOOD	FLAVOR(S)	TEMPERATURE
Apple	Sweet, sour	Cool
Bamboo shoot	Sweet	Cold
Barley	Sweet, salty	Cool
Beef	Sweet	Neutral
Buckwheat	Sweet	Cool
Cayenne	Pungent	Hot
Celery	Sweet, bitter	Cool
Cherry	Sweet	Warm
Chestnut	Sweet	Warm
Chicken	Sweet	Warm
Chickpea	Sweet	Neutral
Chive	Pungent	Warm
Clam (saltwater)	Salty	Cold
Clove	Pungent	Warm
Coriander (seed)	Pungent, sour	Neutral
Cucumber	Sweet	Cool
Eggplant	Sweet	Cool
Fungus (black)	Sweet	Neutral
Garlic	Sweet, pungent, salty	Hot
Ginger (dry)	Pungent	Hot
Ginseng (American)	Sweet, bitter	Neutral
Glutinous rice (sweet rice)	Sweet	Warm
Grapefruit	Sweet, sour	Cold
Horseradish	Pungent	Hot
Kale	Sweet, bitter	Warm
Kuzu	Sweet	Cool

TABLE A.14. STOMACH FOODS (cont.)

FOOD	FLAVOR(S)	TEMPERATURE
Leek	Pungent	Warm
Lentil	Sweet	Neutral
Lettuce	Sweet, bitter	Cool
Licorice	Sweet	Neutral
Mackerel	Sweet	Neutral
Mango	Sweet, sour	Warm
Millet	Sweet, salty	Cool
Mung bean	Sweet	Cool
Mushroom (button)	Sweet	Cool
Mushroom (Chinese black, shiitake)	Sweet	Neutral
Olive	Sweet, sour	Neutral
Oregano	Sweet, pungent	Warm
Papaya	Sweet, bitter	Neutral
Parsley	Pungent, salty, bitter	Warm
Pea (whole, snow)	Sweet	Cool
Peach	Sweet, sour	Warm
Pear	Sweet, sour	Cool
Pepper (black)	Sweet, pungent	Hot
Pepper (white)	Pungent, bitter	Hot
Pollen	Sweet, pungent, salty, sour, bitter	Neutral
Pork	Sweet, salty	Neutral
Potato	Sweet	Neutral
Radish	Sweet, pungent	Cool
Raspberry (leaf)	Sour	Cool
Rice	Sweet	Neutral

TABLE A.14. STOMACH FOODS (cont.)

FOOD	FLAVOR(S)	TEMPERATURE
Sage	Pungent	Warm
Salmon	Sweet	Neutral
Salt	Salty	Cold
Sardine	Sweet, salty	Neutral
Seaweed	Salty	Cold
Sesame oil	Sweet, pungent	Cool
Sorghum	Sweet	Warm
Spinach	Sweet	Cool
Squash	Sweet	Warm
Swiss chard	Sweet	Cool
Taro root	Sweet, pungent	Neutral
Tomato	Sweet, sour	Cold
Trout	Sour	Hot
Turmeric	Pungent, bitter	Warm
Turnip	Sweet, pungent, bitter	Neutral
Vinegar	Sour, bitter	Warm
Water chestnut	Sweet	Cold
Watercress	Pungent, bitter	Warm
Watermelon	Sweet	Cold

TABLE A.15. LUNG FOODS

FOOD	FLAVOR(S)	TEMPERATURE
Almond	Sweet	Neutral
Amaranth	Sweet, bitter	Cool
Aniseed	Sweet, pungent	Warm
Apple	Sweet, sour	Cool
Apricot	Sweet, sour	Neutral
Avocado	Sweet	Cool
Bamboo shoot	Sweet	Cold
Banana	Sweet	Cold
Basil	Sweet, pungent, bitter	Warm
Cantaloupe	Sweet	Cold
Cardamom	Sweet, pungent, bitter	Warm
Carrot	Sweet	Neutral
Cayenne	Pungent	Hot
Chamomile	Sweet, bitter	Cool
Cheese	Sweet, sour	Neutral
Chrysanthemum	Sweet, bitter	Cool
Cinnamon (bark)	Pungent, bitter	Hot
Cinnamon (twig)	Sweet, pungent	Warm
Coriander	Pungent	Warm
Date	Sweet	Warm
Fungus (white)	Sweet	Neutral
Garlic	Sweet, pungent, salty	Hot
Ginger (dry)	Pungent	Hot
Ginger (fresh)	Pungent	Warm
Ginseng (American)	Sweet, bitter	Neutral
Ginseng (Chinese)	Sweet	Warm

TABLE A.15. LUNG FOODS (cont.)

FOOD	FLAVOR(S)	TEMPERATURE
Glutinous rice (sweet rice)	Sweet	Warm
Herring	Sweet	Neutral
Honey	Sweet	Neutral
Horseradish	Pungent	Hot
Kale	Sweet, bitter	Warm
Kumquat	Pungent, sweet	Warm
Leek	Pungent	Warm
Lemon balm	Pungent, sour	Cool
Licorice	Sweet	Neutral
Lima bean	Sweet	Cool
Mandarin orange	Sweet, sour	Cold
Marjoram	Sweet, pungent	Cool
Mulberry	Sweet	Cold
Mushroom (button)	Sweet	Cool
Mustard seed	Pungent	Hot
Nori (dry seaweed)	Sweet, salty	Neutral
Olive	Sweet, sour	Neutral
Onion	Pungent	Warm
Oregano	Sweet, pungent	Warm
Papaya	Sweet, bitter	Neutral
Parsnip	Sweet, pungent	Warm
Peanut (nut and oil)	Sweet	Neutral
Pear	Sweet, sour	Cool
Peppermint	Sweet, pungent	Cool
Persimmon	Sweet	Cold
Pine nut	Sweet	Warm

TABLE A.15. LUNG FOODS (cont.)

FOOD	FLAVOR(S)	TEMPERATURE
Pollen	Sweet, pungent, salty, sour, bitter	Neutral
Pumpkin	Sweet	Neutral
Radish	Sweet, pungent	Cool
Rosemary	Sweet, pungent	Warm
Sage	Pungent	Warm
Savory	Sweet, pungent, bitter	Warm
Scallion	Pungent, bitter	Warm
Sorghum	Sweet	Warm
Strawberry	Sweet, sour	Cool
Swiss chard	Sweet	Cool
Tangerine	Sweet, sour	Cool
Thyme	Pungent, bitter	Warm
Walnut	Sweet	Warm
Water chestnut	Sweet	Cold
Watercress	Pungent, bitter	Warm

TABLE A.16. LARGE INTESTINE FOODS

FOOD	FLAVOR(S)	TEMPERATURE
Avocado	Sweet	Cool
Banana	Sweet	Cold
Beef	Sweet	Neutral
Buckwheat	Sweet	Cool
Chamomile	Sweet, bitter	Cool
Cranberry	Sweet, sour	Cold
Cucumber	Sweet	Cool
Eggplant	Sweet	Cool
Flax	Sweet	Neutral
Fungus (black)	Sweet	Neutral
Honey	Sweet	Neutral
Kuzu	Sweet	Cool
Lemon/lime	Sour	Cold
Licorice	Sweet	Neutral
Mung bean sprout	Sweet	Cold
Mushroom (button)	Sweet	Cool
Nutmeg	Pungent	Warm
Peach	Sweet, sour	Warm
Peanut oil	Sweet	Neutral
Pepper (black)	Sweet, pungent	Hot
Pepper (white)	Pungent, bitter	Hot
Persimmon	Sweet	Cold
Pine nut	Sweet	Warm
Plantain	Sweet	Cold
Pollen	Sweet, pungent, salty, sour, bitter	Neutral
Pumpkin seed	Sweet, bitter	Neutral

TABLE A.16. LARGE INTESTINE FOODS (cont.)

FOOD	FLAVOR(S)	TEMPERATURE
Purslane	Sour	Cold
Rhubarb	Bitter	Cold
Rose hip	Salty, sour	Neutral
Salt	Salty	Cold
Scallion	Pungent, bitter	Warm
Sorghum	Sweet	Warm
Spinach	Sweet	Cool
Swiss chard	Sweet	Cool
Tamarind	Sweet, sour	Cool
Taro root	Sweet, pungent	Neutral
Watercress	Pungent, bitter	Warm
Wheat bran	Sweet	Cool

TABLE A.17. KIDNEY FOODS

FOOD	FLAVOR(S)	TEMPERATURE
Adzuki bean	Sweet, sour	Neutral
Aloe vera	Bitter	Neutral
Asparagus	Sweet, bitter	Cold
Black currant	Sweet, sour	Cool
Celery	Sweet, bitter	Cool
Clam (freshwater)	Sweet, salty	Cold
Cranberry	Sweet, sour	Cold
Cuttlefish	Salty	Neutral
Duck	Sweet	Neutral
Fava bean	Sweet	Neutral
Ginseng (American)	Sweet, bitter	Neutral
Grape	Sweet, sour	Neutral
Kidney bean	Sweet	Neutral
Lemon/lime	Sour	Cold
Lentil	Sweet	Neutral
Licorice	Sweet	Neutral
Marjoram	Sweet, pungent	Cool
Millet	Sweet, salty	Cool
Mulberry	Sweet	Cold
Nettle	Sweet, salty	Cool
Pistachio	Sweet, sour, bitter	Neutral
Salt	Salty	Cold
Seaweed	Salty	Cold
Spinach	Sweet	Cool
Strawberry	Sweet, sour	Cool
Wild Rice	Sweet, sour	Cool

TABLE A.18. BLADDER FOODS

FOOD	FLAVOR(S)	TEMPERATURE
Elderflower	Sweet, pungent, bitter	Cool
Licorice	Sweet	Neutral
Nettle	Sweet, salty	Cool
Parsley	Pungent, salty, bitter	Warm
Pollen	Sweet, pungent, salty, sour, bitter	Neutral
Pomegranate	Sweet, sour	Neutral
Purslane	Sour	Cold
Rose hip	Salty, sour	Neutral
Watermelon	Sweet	Cold
Wax gourd (or winter gourd or winter melon)	Sweet	Cool
Wild rice	Sweet, sour	Cool

TABLE A.19. LIVER FOODS

FOOD	FLAVOR(S)	TEMPERATURE
Adzuki bean	Sweet, sour	Neutral
Artichoke	Sweet, salty, bitter	Cool
Avocado	Sweet	Cool
Blackberry	Sweet, sour	Warm
Black currant	Sweet, sour	Cool
Carrot	Sweet	Neutral
Celery	Sweet, bitter	Cool
Chamomile	Sweet, bitter	Cool
Chinese chive	Pungent	Warm
Chrysanthemum	Sweet, bitter	Cool
Clam (freshwater)	Sweet, salty	Cold
Crab	Salty	Cold
Cumin	Pungent	Warm
Dandelion (leaf and root)	Sweet, salty, bitter	Cold
Dongui	Sweet, pungent	Warm
Eggplant	Sweet	Cool
Elderflower	Sweet, pungent, bitter	Cool
Fenugreek seed	Bitter	Warm
Flax	Sweet	Neutral
Fungus (white)	Sweet	Neutral
Garlic	Sweet, pungent, salty	Hot
Grape	Sweet, sour	Neutral
Hawthorn	Sweet, sour	Warm
Jasmine	Sweet, pungent	Warm
Kumquat	Pungent, sweet	Warm
Leek	Pungent	Warm

TABLE A.19. LIVER FOODS (cont.)

FOOD	FLAVOR(S)	TEMPERATURE
Lemon balm	Pungent, sour	Cool
Lemon/lime	Sour	Cold
Licorice	Sweet	Neutral
Lima bean	Sweet	Cool
Linseed	Sweet	Neutral
Liver (beef)	Sweet	Neutral
Liver (chicken)	Sweet	Warm
Mackerel	Sweet	Neutral
Mulberry	Sweet	Cold
Mussel	Salty	Warm
Nettle	Sweet, salty	Cool
Olive oil	Sweet	Neutral
Peppermint	Sweet, pungent	Cool
Pineapple	Sweet, sour	Hot
Pine nut	Sweet	Warm
Pistachio	Sweet, sour, bitter	Neutral
Pollen	Sweet, pungent, salty, sour, bitter	Neutral
Purslane	Sour	Cold
Radish	Sweet, pungent	Cool
Raspberry	Sweet, sour	Neutral
Rosemary	Sweet, pungent	Warm
Rye	Bitter	Neutral
Saffron	Pungent	Neutral
Sesame (black)	Sweet	Neutral
Shrimp or prawn	Sweet	Warm
Squash (butternut, spaghetti)	Sweet, sour	Warm

TABLE A.19. LIVER FOODS (cont.)

FOOD	FLAVOR(S)	TEMPERATURE
Star anise	Sweet, pungent	Warm
Strawberry	Sweet, sour	Cool
Tomato	Sweet, sour	Cold
Vinegar	Sour, bitter	Warm

TABLE A.20. GALLBLADDER FOODS

FOOD	FLAVOR(S)	TEMPERATURE
Artichoke	Sweet, salty, bitter	Cool
Dandelion (leaf and root)	Sweet, salty, bitter	Cold
Lemon/lime	Sour	Cold
Licorice	Sweet	Neutral
Pollen	Sweet, pungent, salty, sour, bitter	Neutral
Rye	Bitter	Neutral

 Recommended Reading

TAOIST PRACTICES

All of Mantak Chia's books on the Universal Healing Tao practices are based on the Taoist view of the universe, using the yin, yang, and five-element theory. After having read this book and *Inner Alchemy Astrology* and explored your own five-element makeup, you might particularly like to read or reread the following books by Mantak Chia:

The Alchemy of Sexual Energy

Cosmic Fusion, Fusion of the Five Elements, and *Fusion of the Eight Psychic Channels*

Cosmic Nutrition by Mantak Chia and William U. Wei

Craniosacral Chi Kung by Mantak Chia and Joyce Thorn

Emotional Wisdom by Mantak Chia and Dena Saxer (essential entry-level book for understanding Inner Alchemy practices)

Golden Elixir Chi Kung

Healing Light of the Tao

Pi Gu Chi Kung by Mantak Chia and Christine Harkness-Giles

Taoist Cosmic Healing and *Taoist Astral Healing*

The Taoist Soul Body

Taoist Ways to Transform Your Stress into Vitality (essential entry-level book for understanding Inner Alchemy practices)

Wisdom Chi Kung

Some of these are also available in booklet form, shorter but with more anatomical graphics on the practical exercises; they can be instantly downloaded and printed out from the e-shop on the Universal Healing Tao website. You can also find an Inner Alchemy practices class or instructor in your country by looking on the Universal Healing Tao website: **https://www.universaltaoinstructors.com**.

TAOIST OR CHINESE ASTROLOGY

Classical Five Element Chinese Astrology Made Easy by David Twicken
Four Pillars and Oriental Medicine by David Twicken
Spiritual Qi Gong by David Twicken
Treasures of Tao by David Twicken

For a serious study of the subject, understanding the very weighty calculations necessary to do the charting is a necessary step, but if you just want to know a little bit more, then start with:

The Complete Idiot's Guide to Feng Shui, Third Edition by Elizabeth Moran, Master Joseph Yu, and Master Val Biktashev

Although essentially a guide to feng shui (and really the best guide to real feng shui for the general public, highly praised, and read by professionals), the second part of this book is on astrology and is a very good introduction.

CHINESE MEDICINE AND ACUPUNCTURE

(An interesting diversion and a deep, relevant path to healing)

Between Heaven and Earth: A Guide to Chinese Medicine by Harriet Beinfield and Efrem Korngold

The Complete Stems and Branches: Time and Space in Classical Acupuncture by Roisin Golding

Dragon Rises, Red Bird Flies: Psychology & Chinese Medicine by Leon Hammer

The Web That Has No Weaver: Understanding Chinese Medicine by Ted J. Kaptchuk

Wood Becomes Water: Chinese Medicine in Everyday Life by Gail Reichstein

The Yellow Emperor's Classic of Medicine (there are many translations of this ancient Chinese classic)

MASSAGE THERAPIES
(Based on Taoist five-element theory)

Advanced Chi Nei Tsang by Mantak Chia

Chi Nei Ching by Mantak Chia and William U. Wei

Chi Nei Tsang by Mantak Chia

Karsai Nei Tsang by Mantak Chia

Life Pulse Massage: Taoist Techniques for Enhanced Circulation and Detoxification by Mantak Chia and Aisha Sieburth

TAOIST THOUGHT

The Secret and Sublime: Taoist Mysteries and Magic by John Blofeld

The Secret Teachings of the Tao Te Ching by Mantak Chia and Tao Huang

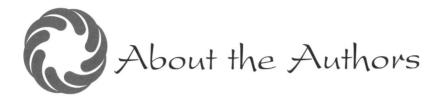 About the Authors

MANTAK CHIA

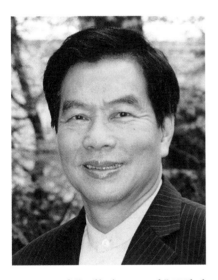

Mantak Chia has been studying the Taoist approach to life since childhood. His mastery of this ancient knowledge, enhanced by his study of other disciplines, has resulted in the development of the Universal Healing Tao system, which is now taught throughout the world.

Mantak Chia was born in Thailand to Chinese parents in 1944. When he was six years old, he learned from Buddhist monks how to sit and "still the mind." While in grammar school he learned traditional Thai boxing, and he soon went on to acquire considerable skill in aikido, yoga, and Tai Chi. His studies of the Taoist way of life began in earnest when he was a student in Hong Kong, ultimately leading to his mastery of a wide variety of esoteric disciplines, thanks to the guidance of several masters, including Master Yi Eng (I Yun) Master Meugi, Master Cheng Yao-Lun, and Master Pan Yu. To better understand the mechanisms behind healing energy, he also studied Western anatomy and medical sciences.

Master Chia has taught his system of healing and energizing practices to tens of thousands of students and trained more than three thousand instructors and practitioners throughout the world. Stemming from his teaching corps, there are established centers for Taoist study and training in many countries around the globe. In June of 1990, he was honored by the International Congress of Chinese Medicine and Qi Gong (Chi Kung), which named him the Qi Gong Master of the Year.

CHRISTINE HARKNESS-GILES

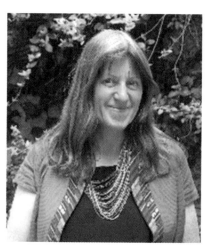

Christine Harkness-Giles is a Universal Healing Tao Instructor and Senior Inner Alchemy Astrology teacher and a feng shui consultant. She lives in London and has been a student of Taoism for many years, studying feng shui, Chinese astrology, and the I Ching, notably with Master Joseph Yu, founder of the Feng Shui Research Centre (FSRC).

Meeting Mantak Chia and learning the Universal Healing Tao practices provided her with the missing link between Taoist knowledge and living its philosophy in today's world. Since then she has been active in organizing Master Chia's teaching visits to Paris, Brussels, and London.

She assisted Master Chia in developing his Inner Alchemy astrology program and now teaches it to the rest of the UHT family, mainly in Berlin and Tao Garden, Thailand. With Master Chia she cowrote *Pi Gu Chi Kung: Inner Alchemy Energy Fasting* and *Inner Alchemy Astrology.*

Inner Alchemy astrology is Mantak Chia's particular form of traditional Chinese astrology. It reveals the five-element makeup of a person and clarifies the role of chi kung and other Taoist techniques in balancing and enhancing one's chi. It can also be usefully combined with five-element nutrition. She uses these techniques with her UHT students and feng shui clients.

The Universal
Healing Tao System
and Training Center

THE UNIVERSAL HEALING TAO SYSTEM

The ultimate goal of Taoist practice is to transcend physical boundaries through the development of the soul and the spirit within the human. That is also the guiding principle behind the Universal Healing Tao, a practical system of self-development that enables individuals to complete the harmonious evolution of their physical, mental, and spiritual bodies. Through a series of ancient Chinese meditative and internal energy exercises, the practitioner learns to increase physical energy, release tension, improve health, practice self-defense, and gain the ability to heal him- or herself and others. In the process of creating a solid foundation of health and well-being in the physical body, the practitioner also creates the basis for developing his or her spiritual potential by learning to tap into the natural energies of the sun, moon, earth, and stars and other environmental forces.

The Universal Healing Tao practices are derived from ancient techniques rooted in the processes of nature. They have been gathered and integrated into a coherent, accessible system for well-being that works directly with the life force, or chi, that flows through the meridian system of the body.

Master Chia has spent years developing and perfecting techniques for teaching these traditional practices to students around the world

187

through ongoing classes, workshops, private instruction, and healing sessions, as well as books and video and audio products. Further information can be obtained at **https://www.universal-tao.com**.

THE UNIVERSAL HEALING TAO TRAINING CENTER

The Tao Garden Resort and Training Center in northern Thailand is the home of Master Chia and serves as the worldwide headquarters for Universal Healing Tao activities. This integrated wellness, holistic health, and training center is situated on eighty acres, surrounded by the beautiful Himalayan foothills near the historic walled city of Chiang Mai. The serene setting includes flower and herb gardens ideal for meditation, open-air pavilions for practicing chi kung, and a health and fitness spa.

The center offers classes year-round, as well as summer and winter retreats. It can accommodate two hundred students, and group leasing can be arranged. For information on courses, books, products, and other resources, see below.

RESOURCES

Universal Healing Tao Center
274 Moo 7, Luang Nua, Doi Saket, Chiang Mai, 50220 Thailand
Tel: (66)(53) 921-200 Fax: (66)(53) 495-852
E-mail: universaltao@universal-tao.com
Website: https://www.universal-tao.com

For information on retreats and the health spa, contact:
Tao Garden Health Spa & Resort
E-mail: info@tao-garden.com, taogarden@hotmail.com
Website: https://www.tao-garden.com

Good Chi • Good Heart • Good Intention . . .
• Good Air and Good Food •

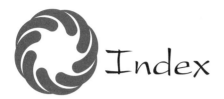 Index

Page numbers in *italics* indicate illustrations and tables.

BOOKS OF RELATED INTEREST

The Eight Immortal Healers
Taoist Wisdom for Radiant Health
by Mantak Chia and Johnathon Dao, M.D. (A.M.), L.Ac.

Cosmic Nutrition
The Taoist Approach to Health and Longevity
by Mantak Chia and William U. Wei

Chi Kung for Prostate Health and Sexual Vigor
A Handbook of Simple Exercises and Techniques
by Mantak Chia and William U. Wei

EMDR and the Universal Healing Tao
An Energy Psychology Approach to Overcoming Emotional Trauma
by Mantak Chia and Doug Hilton

Craniosacral Chi Kung
Integrating Body and Emotion in the Cosmic Flow
by Mantak Chia and Joyce Thom

Healing Light of the Tao
Foundational Practices to Awaken Chi Energy
by Mantak Chia

Chi Self-Massage
The Taoist Way of Rejuvenation
by Mantak Chia

Healing Love through the Tao
Cultivating Female Sexual Energy
by Mantak Chia

INNER TRADITIONS • BEAR & COMPANY
P.O. Box 388
Rochester, VT 05767
1-800-246-8648
www.InnerTraditions.com

Or contact your local bookseller